The Culture of Care

Editors

TIFFANI CHIDUME
KELLIE BRYANT

NURSING CLINICS
OF NORTH AMERICA

www.nursing.theclinics.com

Consulting Editor
BENJAMIN SMALLHEER

March 2024 • Volume 59 • Number 1

ELSEVIER

1600 John F. Kennedy Boulevard • Suite 1800 • Philadelphia, Pennsylvania, 19103-2899

http://www.theclinics.com

NURSING CLINICS OF NORTH AMERICA Volume 59, Number 1
March 2024 ISSN 0029-6465, ISBN-13: 978-0-443-13007-6

Editor: Kerry Holland
Developmental Editor: Isha Singh

Nursing Clinics of North America (ISSN 0029-6465) is published quarterly by Elsevier Inc., 360 Park Avenue South, New York, NY 10010-1710. Months of issue are March, June, September, and December. Periodicals postage paid at New York, NY and additional mailing offices. Subscription price per year is, $168.00 (US individuals), $275.00 (international individuals), $231.00 (Canadian individuals), $100.00 (US and Canadian students), and $135.00 (international students). For institutional access pricing please contact Customer Service via the contact information below. To receive student/resident rate, orders must be accompanied by name of affiliated institution, date of term, and the signature of program/residency coordinator on institution letterhead. Orders will be billed at individual rate until proof of status is received. Foreign air speed delivery is included in all *Clinics* subscription prices. All prices are subject to change without notice. **POSTMASTER:** Send address changes to *Nursing Clinics*, Elsevier Health Sciences Division, Subscription Customer Service, 3251 Riverport Lane, Maryland Heights, MO 63043. **Customer Service: Telephone: 1-800-654-2452** (U.S. and Canada); **1-314-447-8871 (outside U.S. and Canada). Fax: 1-314-447-8029. E-mail: journalscustomerservice-usa@elsevier.com** (for print support) and **journalsonlinesupport-usa@elsevier.com** (for online support).

Nursing Clinics of North America is covered in *EMBASE/Excerpta Medica, MEDLINE/PubMed (Index Medicus), Social Sciences Citation Index, Current Contents, ASCA, Cumulative Index to Nursing, RNdex Top 100,* and Allied Health Literature and International Nursing Index (INI).

Contributors

CONSULTING EDITOR

BENJAMIN SMALLHEER, PhD, RN, ACNP-BC, FNP-BC, CCRN, CNE, FAANP
Assistant Dean, Master of Science in Nursing Program, Associate Professor, Duke
University School of Nursing, Durham, North Carolina, USA

EDITORS

KELLIE BRYANT, DNP, WHNP, CHSE, FAAN
Assistant Dean of Clinical Affairs and Simulation, Associate Professor, Columbia
University School of Nursing, New York, New York, USA

TIFFANI CHIDUME, DNP, RN, CCRN-K, CHSE-A, CHSOS
Associate Clinical Professor, Department of Nursing; Simulation Center Coordinator,
Auburn University College of Nursing, Auburn, Alabama, USA

AUTHORS

BERNICE M. ALSTON, PhD
Director, Student Success, Duke University, Durham, North Carolina, USA

MARY BARZEE, MEd
Grant Manager, Duke University, Durham, North Carolina, USA

MARY A. BEMKER, PhD, PsyS, CNE, RN
Contributing Faculty, Walden University, College of Nursing, Minneapolis, Minnesota, USA

DONNA J. BIEDERMAN, DrPH, MN, RN, CPH, FAAN
Associate Professor, Duke University School of Nursing, Durham, North Carolina, USA

JORDON D. BOSSE, PhD, RN
Assistant Professor, College of Nursing, University of Rhode Island, Providence, Rhode
Island, USA

DEWI BROWN-DEVEAUX, DNP, BS, RN-ONC
Senior Director of Nursing (Patient Engagement and Experience), Department of Nursing,
NYU Langone Health, Brooklyn, New York, USA

LUCINDRA CAMPBELL-LAW, PhD, APRN, ANP, PMHNP-BC
Professor and Divisional Dean of Graduate Programs, University of St. Thomas, Peavy
School of Nursing, Houston, Texas, USA

JOSEPHA CAMPINHA-BACOTE, PhD, MAR, PMHCNS-BC, CTN-A, FAAN, FTNSS
President, Transcultural C.A.R.E. Associates, Blue Ash, Ohio, USA

ETHAN C. CICERO, PhD, RN
Assistant Professor, Emory University, Nell Hodgson Woodruff School of Nursing, Atlanta, Georgia, USA

SEAN P. CONVOY, DNP, PMHNP-BC
Associate Clinical Professor, School of Nursing, Duke University, Durham, North Carolina, USA

JESS DILLARD-WRIGHT, PhD, MA, RN, CNM
Assistant Professor, Elaine Marieb College of Nursing, University of Massachusetts Amherst, Amherst, Massachusetts, USA

DALLAS DUCAR, MSN, RN, APRN, PMHNP-BC, CNL, FAAN
CEO and President, Transhealth, Chelsea, Massachusetts, USA

KIMBERLEY ENNIS, DNP, APRN-BC
Senior Director of Nursing, Patient Engagement and Experience, Department of Nursing, NYU Langone Health, Site Lead for Nursing and Patient Care Services, Yonkers, New York, USA

JULIA GAMBLE, MSN, NP
Advance Practice Provider, Duke Outpatient Clinic, Durham, North Carolina, USA

ASHLEY GRAHAM-PEREL, EDD, RN, NPD-BC, MEDSURG-BC, CNE
Interim Director of the Office of Diversity and Cultural Affairs, Assistant Professor of Nursing, Columbia University School of Nursing, Jamaica, New York, USA

MITCHELL HEFLIN, MD, MHS
Associate Dean and Director, Center for Interprofessional Education and Care (IPEC), Duke University, Professor of Medicine, Division of Geriatrics, Duke University School of Medicine, Senior Fellow, Aging Center at Duke, Medical Director, Geriatric Evaluation and Treatment Clinic Duke University School of Medicine, Durham, North Carolina, USA

UNDI HOFFLER, PhD
Director, Research Compliance and Technology Transfer, Division of Research and Sponsored Programs, North Carolina State University Raleigh, North Carolina, USA

LINDA JOHANSON, EDD, MS(N), RN
Core Faculty, Walden University, College of Nursing, Minneapolis, Minnesota, USA

TINISHA LAMBETH, DNP, NNP-BC
Assistant Professor, Department of Academic Nursing, Wake Forest University, School of Medicine, Winston-Salem, North Carolina, USA

AMY S. D. LEE, DNP, ARNP, WHNP-BC
Clinical Associate Professor, Capstone College of Nursing, The University of Alabama Tuscaloosa, Alabama, USA

LUCI NEW, DNP, CRNA
Assistant Professor, Wake Forest University, School of Medicine, Department of Academic Nursing, Winston-Salem, North Carolina, USA

HEATHER O'DONOHUE, MS, BSN, RN
Registered Nurse, Medicine II Novant Health New Hanover Regional Medical Center, Wilmington, North Carolina, USA

BLANCA IRIS PADILLA, PhD, MBA, APRN, MSN, FNP-BC, FAANP
Associate Professor, Duke University School of Nursing, Duke University Health System, Durham, North Carolina, USA

ANGELA RICHARD-EAGLIN, DNP, MSN, FNP-BC, CNE, FAANP
Associate Professor, Associate Dean for Equity, Yale School of Nursing, West Haven, Connecticut, USA

CHRISTINE RODRIGUEZ, DNP, APRN, FNP-BC, MDIV, MA
Assistant Professor, Assistant Dean of Simulation and Clinical Innovation, Yale School of Nursing, Yale University, Orange, Connecticut, USA

MAYRA RODRIGUEZ, PhD, MPH
Discipline Chair for Epidemiology, Community and Public Health, and Preventive Medicine, Edward Via College of Osteopathic Medicine Auburn, Auburn, Alabama, USA

DEBRA H. SULLIVAN, PhD, MSN, RN, CNE, COI
Senior Core Faculty, Walden University, College of Nursing, Minneapolis, Minnesota, USA

JULIE ANNE THOMPSON, PhD
Health Data Analyst, Duke University, Consulting Associate, School of Nursing, Duke University, Durham, North Carolina, USA

TERRY THROCKMORTON, PhD, RN
Faculty, University of St. Thomas, Peavy School of Nursing, Houston, Texas, USA

PATTI P. URSO, PhD, APRN, ANP-BC, FNP, CNE
Specialization Coordinator, Nursing Education Walden University, College of Nursing, Minneapolis, Minnesota, USA

KATILYA S. WARE, PhD, RN
Assistant Professor, Auburn University College of Nursing, Auburn, Alabama, USA

MICHELLE WEBB, DNP, MSN, RN, CHPCA
Assistant Clinical Professor, Duke University School of Nursing, Durham, North Carolina, USA

RICHARD WESTPHAL, PhD, RN, PMHCNS-BC, PMHNP-BC, FAAN
School of Nursing, Charlottesville, VA United States Professor, Family, Community and Mental Health Systems, University of Virginia Auburn, Alabama, USA

COURTNEY H. WILLIAMS, BSc (Psychology)
Graduate Research Assistant, Auburn University College of Nursing, School of Nursing, Charlottesville, Virginia, USA

Contents

With the introduction of more complex health conditions and the changing landscape of the healthcare infrastructure, burnout is increasingly becoming a crisis for the nursing profession and for the public. Recruitment in nursing must consider the concept of a nurturing environment as a key driver of sustainability within the profession. Human beings cannot flourish in hostile and unwelcoming environments. Failure to thrive in nursing is a real phenomenon that is driven by multiple factors, including incivility, workplace bullying, and lack of support. Mitigation requires intentional, strategic interventions toward building nurturing environments in education and practice for the next generation of nurses.

Nursing academicians are positioned at a critical juncture to mold the future generations of nursing with the skills of cultural humility, starting with fostering humility in the classroom. The dynamic culture of nursing education, with consideration of the diversity of nursing students and faculty, commands attention before the exploration of what is taught about the culture of patients. Classroom cultural humility must become the "brave space" of nursing academia. This is possible with strategic approaches and revisiting the history of the culture of nursing education before trying to shape its future.

True holistic care implies an in-depth assessment and understanding of patient needs based on their physical, social, psychological, and spiritual makeup. These parameters are affected by their native culture as well as their adopted culture. The culture of a patient is composed of beliefs, values, and lifestyles. Understanding the general elements of specific cultures and religions can provide a basis for more insightful inquiry with patients regarding their preferences in health care. This article includes basic beliefs and practices related to 5 patient populations.

describing techniques to overcome institutional-level challenges that may hinder a nurse's ability to establish gender-affirming therapeutic relationships with TNGE people. The authors also provide strategies that nurses can use to improve their health care organization and interprofessional collaborative practice to create psychologically and physically safe health care spaces for TNGE people.

demonstrate compassion toward both employees and patients. This article explores the significance of creating and supporting a culture of care for both patients and employees in health care organizations. Finally, the article identifies prevalent practices that contribute to a culture of care.

All in health care are at risk of involvement in adverse events. Oftentimes, the health care worker manifests physical, psychological, and professional effects and this is referred to as the second-victim phenomenon. Unmitigated recovery of a second victim can contribute to absenteeism, turnover intentions, burnout, and loss of joy and meaning in work. The preferred method of support among health care workers is a respected peer to provide emotional support. Health care organizations can contribute to a second victim's recovery by providing a culture of safety and diverse resources based on the needs of the individual.

NURSING CLINICS

SERIES OF RELATED INTEREST

Advances in Family Practice Nursing
www.advancesinfamilypracticenursing.com

THE CLINICS ARE AVAILABLE ONLINE!
Access your subscription at:
www.theclinics.com

Foreword

Bring Discussions on the Culture of Care in Nursing to the Forefront

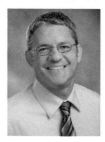

Benjamin Smallheer, PhD, RN, ACNP-BC, FNP-BC, CCRN, CNE, FAANP
Consulting Editor

It is often said, "*nursing is a caring profession*," But what exactly does that mean? Jean Watson, in the *Theory of Human Caring*,[1] defines caring as values, a will, and a commitment to care, knowledge, caring actions, and consequences. However, there is more to caring than such a sterile definition. How caring is expressed will vary greatly by the nature of the situation at hand. The loss of a child will elicit a very different response than failing a nursing school pharmacology exam. An executive in the C-suite of a major health system will spend a different amount of time asking about how things are at home than a daycare aide on a preschool playground. Feelings of loneliness will be investigated by a grandparent with much more intention than that of an astringed neighbor who lives at the end of the cul-de-sac.

Let's raise the complexity one more notch. Rather than considering what caring "looks" like, consider how caring behaves, what caring believes, the values of caring, and accepted mechanisms of caring…without having to think about them. When these aspect points are combined, we now have approached an unfamiliar concept: the culture of caring. Culture is most associated with characteristics of an individual's identity, such as food, clothing, religious practices, and locations of origin.[2] Associating culture with caring practices, however, presents a new notion that is impacted by an extensive number of factors. Settling into this exploration and investigation brings us to an intersection of global identity and individualized health care.

This issue of *Nursing Clinics of North America* takes the reader on a guided exploration across academia, religion, interprofessional collaborations, psych-mental health, housing instability, gender affirmation, health inequity, social injustice, and the collateral damage experienced by those in nursing traumatized by unanticipated adverse events (second-victim phenomenon). This issue represents a journey of bravery and

Nurs Clin N Am 59 (2024) xiii–xiv
https://doi.org/10.1016/j.cnur.2023.11.012
0029-6465/24/© 2023 Published by Elsevier Inc.

vulnerability taken by man but spoken about so seldom. This new journey is focusing forward on how to advance aspects of caring for those whose voices have been silenced or not been granted a place at the table. We move into this space to support our friends, colleagues, family, those we don't know, or maybe even those we do not particularly like. We invite you to explore with us and set your own compass on *The Culture of Care*.

Benjamin Smallheer, PhD, RN, ACNP-BC, FNP-BC, CCRN, CNE, FAANP
Duke University School of Nursing
307 Trent Drive
DUMC Box 3322
Durham, NC 27710, USA

E-mail address:
benjamin.smallheer@duke.edu

REFERENCES

1. Watson J Nursing. human science and human care. New York: National League for Nursing; 1988.
2. Patient Safety Network (PSNet). Cultural competence and patient safety. Agency for Healthcare Research and Quality. 2019. Available at: https://psnet.ahrq.gov/perspective/cultural-competence-and-patient-safety. Accessed November 15, 2023.

Preface

Variations of the Culture of Care

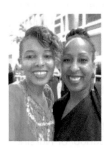

Tiffani Chidume,
DNP, RN, CCRN-K,
CHSE-A, CHSOS and
Kellie Bryant, DNP,
WHNP, CHSE, FAAN
Editors

In the ever-evolving landscape of health care, understanding and embracing the culture of various populations has become an indispensable facet of nursing practice. The field of nursing has undergone a profound transformation in recent years, transcending its traditional boundaries to become a global endeavor. As nurses, we find ourselves caring for individuals from diverse backgrounds, each with their unique beliefs, traditions, and values. The fabric of health care is intricately woven with the threads of culture, and our ability to provide compassionate and effective care hinges on our mastery of what we term "the culture of care."

Within these pages, we will embark on a journey through the rich tapestry of cultural diversity, acknowledging that culture encompasses more than just ethnicity—it encompasses gender, socioeconomic status, religion, sexual orientation, and countless other dimensions of identity. We will delve into the intricacies of cultural humility, transcultural nursing, and the profound ways in which culture influences the health and well-being of our patients.

As nurses, we are entrusted with the responsibility of being advocates, caregivers, and educators. By recognizing and embracing the culture of our patients, we empower ourselves to deliver care that is not only clinically competent but also culturally sensitive and respectful. A culture of care in nursing includes providing a holistic approach to patient-centered care that emphasizes cultural humility and respects the diverse backgrounds of our patients. This approach fosters trust and enhances patient-provider relationships that will ultimately lead to promoting health equity.

This issue of *Nursing Clinics of North America* serves as a beacon of knowledge, a source of inspiration, and a forum for critical reflection as we explore the complexities of "the culture of care." We invite you, the dedicated nurse, the curious student, and

Nurs Clin N Am 59 (2024) xv–xvi
https://doi.org/10.1016/j.cnur.2023.11.001
0029-6465/24/© 2023 Published by Elsevier Inc.

nursing.theclinics.com

the passionate advocate for health care equity, to join us in this exploration of "the culture of care." Together, we will celebrate the diversity that enriches our profession and, through knowledge, compassion, and understanding, strive to provide care that respects and embraces the cultures of those we serve.

May the words and experiences shared in these pages inspire you to embark on your own journey of cultural discovery and competence and may they reinforce the essential truth that in nursing, as in life, embracing the culture of care is not just important—it is fundamental to our mission and our calling.

Tiffani Chidume, DNP, RN, CCRN-K, CHSE-A, CHSOS
Auburn University College of Nursing
710 South Donahue Drive
Auburn, AL 35849, USA

Kellie Bryant, DNP, WHNP, CHSE, FAAN
Columbia University School of Nursing
560 West 168th Street
New York, NY 10032, USA

E-mail addresses:
tlc0045@auburn.edu (T. Chidume)
Kdb2146@cumc.columbia.edu (K. Bryant)

Strategies for Developing a Nurturing Environment for the next Generation of Nurses

Angela Richard-Eaglin, DNP, MSN, FNP-BC, CNE[a],*,
Michelle Webb, DNP, MSN, RN, CHPCA[b]

KEYWORDS

- Nurturing • Incivility • Cultural intelligence • Mindfulness • Reconciliation • Culture
- Ethics

KEY POINTS

- A nurturing environment across venues in nursing can promote allegiance to and sustainability in the profession.
- Incivility and bullying thwart efforts to nurture the next generation of nurses.
- The American Nurses Association Code of Ethics holds nurses accountable for upholding the professional standards of nursing through advocacy for self and others.
- Intentional strategies such as cultural intelligence, mindfulness, role modeling, and truth and reconciliation can support building and maintaining a nurturing environment.

INTRODUCTION

The crux of nursing is built upon caring and compassion. Traditionally, nursing education around these concepts has emphasized caring and compassion for patients and families, while neglecting espousal of a culture of caring in the learning environment. To change this narrative, it is imperative that nurse educators facilitate culture shifts that prioritize and normalize a broad array of cultural needs among learners. Creating an optimal learning environment challenges nurse educators to not only consider demographically designated needs, but to also consider diverse abilities among learners. While diversity has become both a buzzword and a bad word for some, advancing health equity requires nursing and the larger healthcare community to recognize its significance and refute those narratives. In its broadest sense, diversity refers to all differences among individuals and groups of people.[1] Authentically embracing these differences engenders trust-building, an essential element of

[a] Yale School of Nursing, PO Box 27399, West Haven, CT 06477, USA; [b] Duke University School of Nursing, 3113 Pearson Siegler Building, Durham, NC 27710, USA
* Corresponding author.
E-mail address: angela.richard-eaglin@yale.edu

Nurs Clin N Am 59 (2024) 1–9
https://doi.org/10.1016/j.cnur.2023.11.002
0029-6465/24/© 2023 Elsevier Inc. All rights reserved.

nursing.theclinics.com

genuine relationships. These relationships are significant first steps for in-the-moment mentoring processes for nurses, but also for inspiring them to serve as mentors for future generations. The collateral result exudes a culture of nurturing. Diversity in all forms is critical to fostering nurturing environments that catalyze innovations in educational and clinical settings. Additionally, diversity is critical to achieving a representative workforce and to advancing health equity.

The American Association of Colleges of Nursing is calling for expanding diversity in the workforce; therefore, the learning environment must shift from the traditional physical environments and pedagogical methodologies to one that is genuinely representative of a multiplicity of cultures not only visually, but through cultivation of authentic and deep connections with every individual and group within the space. The return on investment is equitable outcomes for everyone. It is imperative that the culture shifts begin in the classroom for translation to practice to occur. New traditions and new ways of thinking and being are critical to this transformation. The nexus of these is role modeling and accountability. This paper will provide the historical context for the importance of nurturing and highlight strategies that can rewrite the narrative for the next generation of nurses.

CULTURE OF PROFESSIONAL NURSING

Nursing is a humanitarian profession, which begets adoption of the humanitarian principles: service, mercy, compassion, and respect for human life and dignity.[2] The American Nurses Association (ANA) describes the Code of Ethics as "the profession's non-negotiable ethical standard" Figure and as nursing's interpretation of its commitment to society.[3] Even so, there is a history and ongoing presence of bullying and incivility among nurses. A systematic review and meta-synthesis of nursing students' experiences with incivility highlight the adage that "nurses eat their young".[4] The review reiterated reports of bullying and disparate treatment, largely rooted in biases related to gender, scholastic performance, socioeconomic status, and affinity bias.[4] Examples of affinity bias in nursing include demonstrated or communicated preferences to teach, precept, and mentor students of a certain race/ethnicity, age or gender. Incivility in nursing is not only prevalent in the learning environment, but it also persists in the behavior. Students and other nurses often live what they learn. Failure to nurture and burnout are broad consequences of incivility that compromise efforts at high-quality care, threaten patient safety, and ultimately, perpetuate suboptimal health outcomes.[5] Additionally, incivility and bullying thwart efforts to nurture the next generation of nurses. The most detrimental manifestations of incivility in individual nurses are low self-confidence and physiologic stress responses.[5] The most common physiologic stress responses are increased risk of chronic physical conditions such as hypertension and cardiac disease, as well as mental health conditions, such as anxiety and depression.[5]

The ANA Code of Ethics for Nurses emphasizes the standards of professional behaviors. Provision one of the ANA Code of Ethics states that "A fundamental principle that underlies all nursing practice is respect for the inherent dignity, worth, unique attributes, and human rights of all individuals". [3 (p.1)] It further asserts that nurses in all areas of practice must comprehensively consider every aspect of each person's culture.[3 (p.1)] Nursing practice does not simply apply to patient care; therefore, it is imperative that incivility in nursing becomes a zero-tolerance mandate. Provision 6 states that nurses must individually and collectively institute and sustain an environment of ethical comportment.[3] In essence, this provision obliges nurses to prioritize a safe milieu that is favorable to high-quality care. Provision 9 holds nurses accountable for pledging and demonstrating professional values, maintaining professional integrity, and incorporating social justice principles in policies and practice.[3]

Practices of incivility and bullying are adversarial to the ANA Code of Ethics for Nurses, but this pattern continues despite the ANA positing that adherence to these standards is not optional. They must be adhered to with consistency. As a foundational means to understanding the importance of ethical comportment, experienced nurses in every facet of the profession are obligated to subscribe to each type of ethics as described by the ANA: (1) metaethics addresses the "why" certain behaviors are necessary, (2) normative ethics promotes understanding of the "what" of human behaviors, and (3) applied ethics defines the "how" in actuating the expected behaviors.[3] Understanding the cause and effect of the behaviors of nurses and the implications of failure to nurture is a prerequisite for developing and operationalizing the norms and expectations of the professional nurse.[3] The "why of metaethics is tied to outcomes, outcomes for the next generation of nurses, patients, families, organizations, communities, and populations.[3] Normative ethics aids in establishing shared practice standards that influence the professional culture.[3] These norms delineate expected behaviors and consequences.[3] Applied ethics is demonstrative and includes intentions and impact, role modeling, and advocacy.[3]

Many professional organizations boast the mission of *Better Health for All People* and envision closing disparity gaps through endorsement of diversity and demarginalization initiatives. Actualizing these standards and goals means that rigidity and a provincial perspective can no longer be the guideposts for nursing education and practice. Many are hyper-focused on expected sociocultural and other demographic changes within the general population; however, this has not been a priority strategy for developing approaches for engagement with the next generation of nurses. Historically, the person-centric needs of marginalized and underrepresented students have not been accounted for in the learning environment. Norms have been centered around Eurocentrism and ableism, which has forced assimilation, created exclusion, and limited efforts to embrace difference and cultivate holistic and nurturing learning and work environments. Consequently, many nurses have not reaped the benefits that role modeling these behaviors can have on outcomes that transcend the learning environment. Impartiality and equitable care for all humans is mandated by the ANA Code of Ethics.[3] Empathy, caring, and compassion are the foundations from which humans can gain the ability to embrace difference. A strategic process is imperative for the transition to be effective and sustainable. A re-envisioned version of the nursing process may be ideal.

THE NURTURING ENVIRONMENT AND ITS IMPACT

The nurturing environment should transcend healthcare across venues and systems, from the classroom to the boardroom. While numerous sources[6–8] are available to guide the creation of a nurturing environment, the ANA Code of Ethics should underpin development of person-centric learning environments to transform the historical practices that did not previously consider a multiplicity of cultures and norms. The Future of Nursing 2020 to 2030 Report recommends organizational accountability and responsibility for protecting the well-being of nurses by establishing ethically sound and psychologically safe workplaces that are devoid of bullying and incivility.[9] Nursing practice encompasses every aspect of the profession, including clinical practice, teaching, leadership, scholarship, and research.

The experience in a nurturing environment is not characterized by mere *tolerance* of differences but by *acceptance* and embracing a person's total humanity. Tolerance implies superficiality and forceful interaction or putting up with something or someone. Acceptance implies sincerity in embracing the sum of the individual, as well as of its parts. This level of authenticity is both encouraged and affirmed through nurturing. The resultant benefaction is a sense of well-being and belonging that promotes thriving rather than simply surviving in an environment. A nurturing environment fosters an equitable, inclusive experience in the learning space and in practice environments. Every individual has equal access to opportunities that address their unique socio-cultural needs, is treated equitably by all members of the learning and practice community, and feels valued and supported by their peers, mentors, and supervisors. The diverse multicultural needs of nurses must be conspicuously and strategically addressed to co-create and promulgate a nurturing environment that challenges broader narratives imbued by cognitive biases and furthers critical literacy.[10] The impact of a nurturing learning environment is determined by the student experience, transfers to professional nursing practice, and ultimately impacts the experience of populations being served.

STRATEGIES FOR CREATING AND SUSTAINING A NURTURING ENVIRONMENT

Nurturing, much like mentoring, supports and encourages growth and development of others.[10] A nurturing environment across venues in nursing can promote allegiance to and sustainability in the profession. The creation of a sustainable nurturing environment requires strategic planning and intentionality with a focus on developing cultural intelligence (CQ), building social agency, providing positive role-modeling, and preventing harm and re-traumatization. This approach is critical for those whose education and professional practice environments may have been marked by cultural insensitivity, incivility, antagonism, or career trauma events[11]; environments that can fail to honor and value diverse cultural values preferences and lived experiences. Operationalizing the humanitarian principles that the nursing profession espouses begins with providing trust-building experiences for all learners and practicing nurses. Preparing new graduate nurses for entry into professional practice vis-a-vis a nurturing learning environment will support the development of personal resilience and professional growth and development at all career stages. Building and sustaining a nurturing environment requires strategies that (1) foster the development of critical literacy and CQ, (2) intrapersonal and interpersonal well-being within the learning community, and (3) apply principles of truth and reconciliation to promote a healthy, just culture. Role modeling should be used as an overarching strategy to diffuse the knowledge, skills, and attitudes needed to create and sustain a nurturing environment.

CRITICAL LITERACY

Critical literacy requires the ability to actively read and move beyond simply absorbing information. The critically literate individual questions biases, opinions, and motivations with analytical regard. Critical literacy broadens perspective to include consideration of the context of the work. Curiosity about other perspectives that may be misinterpreted or unapparent is inspired prompting questions such as, *what is the intended message of a person's communications?* and *what are other perspectives on this issue or situation?*[12] Critical literacy aids in appreciation and openness to multiple perspectives. Lewison and colleagues (2002) list 4 dimensions of critical literacy[8].

1. Disrupting the commonplace
2. Interrogating multiple viewpoints
3. Focusing on sociopolitical issues

4. Taking action and promoting social justice.[12, (p.382)]

Critical literacy development practices can be transformative. For nurse educators and nurse leaders managing increasingly diverse constituencies, critical literacy offers tools to engage different viewpoints and life experiences that may diverge greatly from their own. It is this ability to engage that contributes to a learning environment that truly "nurtures" and promotes an optimal learning experience.[12]

Using Counter-narratives to Develop Critical Literacy

Counter-narratives are stories that recount the experiences and perspectives of those who are historically oppressed, excluded, or silenced.[13] The use of counter-narratives validates the experiences and perspectives of historically marginalized groups and can be used to disrupt and challenge dominant social and cultural narratives that impede the actualization of a nurturing environment. Counter-narratives serve to frame and reframe personal narratives as valuable and necessary sources of knowledge in classrooms and in practice settings to promote equity and the development of critical literacy.[14] In an increasingly multicultural environment of nursing education and practice, words truly have power and "our stories are told using words and language habits that often imbue bias about people's intent or specific actions".[15,(para4)] In the learning environment and in the workplace, counter-narrative perspectives can be introduced through readings, lectures, case studies and multimedia, as well as guide the selection of guest speakers and presenters who bring diverse perspectives.[15] As opportunities to engage with counter-narratives are presented, nurses in every role can center the voices and experiences that would otherwise go unheard. Mastery of the use of the counter-narrative as a tool for development of deep learning and understanding can assist with strategic presentation of stories that enhance the nurturing environment, build CQ, and enable looking beyond the story. This process helps to uncover the assumptions behind dominant narratives and co-create new narratives that are inclusive of diverse perspectives and truths.[14] The end result informs a sense of value for all learners and nurses.

CULTURAL INTELLIGENCE

The CQ framework can bolster capacity to embrace difference and broaden individual perspectives. Cultural intelligence is the ability to function effectively in culturally diverse environments.[16,17] Expanding on that definition, CQ provides individuals and groups with tools that foster open mindedness and perspective building beyond each person's unique lived experience. In turn, people develop the skills to automatically consider a multiplicity of norms and abilities, rather than relying solely on their personal values and preferences to guide interactions. Cultural intelligence (CQ) and emotional intelligence (EI) are 2 distinctly different yet related concepts. Emotional intelligence is a set of skills needed to assess, regulate, and influence emotion in self and others[18] and is essential to the development of CQ. However, EI is culturally conditioned creating the need for CQ to elevate the capability to work effectively in multicultural contexts. Achieving 4 interconnected capabilities constitute CQ: (1) Drive, (2) knowledge, (3) strategy, and (4) action.[16,17] Cultural intelligence drive is the desire to interact in multicultural environments; CQ knowledge is comprehension of cultural similarities and differences; CQ strategy is the process of analyzing cultural differences to plan for transcultural interaction; CQ action involves acknowledging personal norms, accepting the norms of other people and adapting, rather than trying to impose our norms on other people.[16,17] Building CQ may be best achieved with critical self-analysis and awareness as a first step. Proficiency in CQ broadens perspective and impels empathy and compassion through deep understanding and acceptance of difference. Consequently, people with high levels of CQ are more apt to advocate for and facilitate nurturing.

MINDFULNESS-BASED INTERVENTIONS AND PRACTICES

Regardless of the area of practice, that is, clinical, research, academia, or leadership, nurses quickly learn the importance of multitasking as a means to successfully perform the job. Competing demands in learning environments and in the workplace make it difficult to be self-aware, and in turn, nurses may engage in behaviors that are not conducive to building a culture of collegiality and nurturing. While some nurses knowingly subscribe to hazing students and their colleagues, oftentimes, aberrant behaviors toward others are unintentional. Provision 5 of the ANA Code of Ethics obliges nurses to prioritize self-care as a means of maintaining personal disposition, integrity, competence, and professional growth and development.[3] As such, nurses who adhere to this principle through intentionality of self-preservation will likely experience less burnout, and perhaps, be less likely to threaten a nurturing environment. As previously noted in the section of this paper on the historical culture of nursing, incivility and bullying remain commonplace within the profession. So, while we have been aware of the problem, very little has been done to intervene and change the narrative.

Defined as the intrinsic ability to be fully present in the moment, self-aware, and peripherally aware, mindfulness is one intervention that may help dissuade nurses from engaging in untoward behaviors.[19,20] Although mindfulness is inherent, accessing it is not always second nature.[15,16] An integrative review by Schuman-Olivier and colleagues[20] describes the influence of mindfulness on behavior change, including improvement in mental and physical health behaviors.[20]

The awareness that is produced by mindfulness can serve as a powerful tool to aid in self-regulation of behaviors. The ability to observe occurrences within our minds not only improves all areas of personal performance, but also increases acuity. This increased insight influences the expansion of personal perspective and the ability to be more aware and concerned with the well-being of others.[20,21] Effective application of mindfulness improves personhood and interpersonal acumen, thus enhancing the nurses' ability to adhere to the ANA principles of self-care and advocacy for others.[3] Studies show that mindfulness-based interventions and practices contribute to improved outlook, increased job satisfaction, and decreased burnout.[20,21] It stands to reason that resulting outcomes would positively influence a nurturing environment.

APPLYING JUST CULTURE PRINCIPLES AND PRINCIPLES OF TRUTH AND RECONCILIATION

The presence of a just culture is a hallmark of a nurturing environment and a concept with analogous application to both the academic learning environment and the professional nursing practice learning environment. Those engaged in the study of nursing and those who currently practice as licensed nurses need a safe haven for learning from clinical and interpersonal mistakes. Just culture is a concept linked to systems thinking that emphasizes that mistakes are principally the result of faulty organizational cultures and systems, and therefore the appropriate first response is not to 'blame the individual' but to interrogate the system to determine accountability and responsibility for learning and improvement.[22] One of the norms of just culture is to ensure that medical errors are examined through a lens of justice to ensure that these events do not lead to a "second victim syndrome" and immutable professional and personal trauma[19] Nursing professionals, as members of the most trusted profession, often expect perfection of themselves, and this prevailing tendency has historically been communicated directly and indirectly to aspiring students of the practice.[23] The commitment to foster a more nurturing, empowering practice and learning environment is a paradigm shift from this historical cultural norm. When mistakes that harm or have the potential for harm are made within the learning community, adopting a just culture approach and applying principles of truth and reconciliation can restore a healthy, nurturing learning milieu and prevent future and deeper harm. Reconciliation has been aptly described as "a process of healing of relationships that requires public truth sharing, apology, and commemoration that acknowledge and redress past harms" [24 (p.3)] This concept has an origin in the work of governmental and other justice advocacy initiatives. These principles have been applied to bring about justice for historically marginalized and oppressed peoples.[22–24] At first glance, it may seem far-reaching to apply these principles to nursing learning and practice communities. However, the process that is needed to restore trust, promote social agency and the nurturing spirit essential to a positive learning experience has similitude. If nurses are to flourish in prescribed environments, the relevance of these principles to the restoration and protection of perceived psychologically safe spaces must be considered.

SUMMARY

Recruitment in nursing must consider the concept of a nurturing environment as a key driver of sustainability within the profession. A learning environment is more than just a classroom—it is a space where learners of all types feel safe and supported in their pursuit of knowledge and professional growth and development. What happens in the learning environment critically matters. Just as in the notion that *children live what they learn*, the same often holds true for nursing students, many of whom are impressionable and eager to learn. Therefore, nurse educators bear a huge responsibility to role model what empathy, compassion, and respect for human life and dignity should look like, beginning with the way they personally treat students and transcend to protecting and supporting students across all learning spheres. Human beings cannot flourish in hostile and unwelcoming environments. Failure to thrive in nursing is a real phenomenon that is driven by multiple factors, including incivility, workplace bullying, and lack of support. Mitigation requires intentional, strategic interventions toward building nurturing environments in education and practice for the next generation of nurses.

Nursing students and practicing professional nurses need and deserve the outputs that result from carefully and strategically designed, nurturing spaces. Increasingly complex health conditions and the changing landscape of healthcare systems and care delivery have exacerbated the experiences of mental fatigue to a burnout crisis. Recognizing and responding to the need to nurture is crucial in fortifying the health of the profession and the health of the public. As our profession emerges from an ongoing and ever-evolving global pandemic, the critical lesson of the importance of prioritizing the health and well-being of nursing students and professionals has been permanently imprinted in the collective wisdom of the profession, key stakeholders in the healthcare system in the United States, and the global community of citizens who need a resilient and hopeful workforce of nurses. Ultimately, the learning environment determines the student's experience, transfers to professional nursing practice, and in the final analysis, impacts the experience and outcomes for the patient populations being served.

CLINICS CARE POINTS

- Peer advocacy and support are essential in limiting burnout associated with the inherent stress of nursing, especially clinical nursing.
- Role modeling self-care is a critical component of nurturing the next generation of nurses.
- Senior leaders must invest in taking steps to break the cycle of incivility in nursing to sustain the profession.
- Mentoring must become a standardized and ongoing operationalized expectation of professional nursing.

DISCLOSURE

The authors do not have commercial or financial conflicts of interests or funding sources.

REFERENCES

1. Merriam-Webster: America's Most Trusted Dictionary. Accessed August 25, 2023. https://www.merriam-webster.com/.
2. Bernard V. The humanitarian ethos in action. Int Rev Red Cross 2015; 97(897–898):7–18.
3. Code of Ethics for Nurses. ANA. Published October 26, 2017. Accessed August 25, 2023. https://www.nursingworld.org/practice-policy/nursing-excellence/ethics/code-of-ethics-for-nurses/.
4. Zhu Z, Xing W, Lizarondo L, et al. Nursing students' experiences with faculty incivility in the clinical education context: a qualitative systematic review and meta-synthesis. BMJ Open 2019;9(2):e024383.
5. Kim Y, Lee E, Lee H. Association between workplace bullying and burnout, professional quality of life, and turnover intention among clinical nurses. PLoS One 2019;14(12):e0226506 [published correction appears in PLoS One. 2020 Jan 16;15(1):e0228124].
6. AACN Standards for Establishing and Sustaining Healthy Work Environments: A Journey to Excellence. Published online 2016. www.aacn.org.
7. American Nurses Association. Professional Issues Panel on Incivility, Bullying, and, Workplace Violence. Position Paper. Published online July 22, 2015. Accessed October 23, 2023. https://www.nursingworld.org/.
8. National League for Nursing Healthful Work Environment Toolkit. Published online 2018. nln.org.
9. Flaubert JL, Le Menestrel S, Williams DR, et al, editors. National Academies of Sciences, Engineering, and Medicine; National academy of medicine; committee on the future of nursing 2020–2030. The future of nursing 2020-2030: charting a path to achieve health equity. . Washington (DC): National Academies Press (US); 2021.
10. O'Brien EM, O' Donnell C, Murphy J, et al. Intercultural readiness of nursing students: An integrative review of evidence examining cultural competence educational interventions. Nurse Educ Pract 2021;50:102966.
11. Pearson E. Career Trauma Is a Real Thing. Here's How to Recognize and Recover From It. Entrepreneur, 2021. Accessed August 23, 2023. https://www.entrepreneur.com/living/career-trauma-is-a-real-thing-heres-how-to-recognize-and/385839.

12. Lewison M, Flint AS, Sluys KV, et al. Taking on critical literacy: The journey of new-comers and novices. Lang Arts 2002;79(2):382–92.
13. Bergen JK, Hantke SU, Denis V. Contemporary challenges and approaches in anti-racist teacher education. In: Tierney RJ, Rizvi F, Ercikan K, editors. International encyclopedia of education. Fourth Edition. Elsevier; 2023. p. 414–26.
14. Miller R, Liu K, Ball AF. Critical Counter-Narrative as Transformative Methodology for Educational Equity. Rev Res Educ 2020;44(1):269–300.
15. Bamberg M. Master and counter narratives Same facts – different stories. RO 2021;(122).
16. Earley PC, Ang S. Cultural intelligence: individual interactions across cultures. Stanford University Press; 2003.
17. Livermore D. Cultural intelligence. In: LearnCQ.com. 2022. Available at: https://www.learncq.com/credentials/. Accessed January 20, 2022.
18. Salovey P, Mayer JD. Emotional Intelligence. Imagin, Cognit Pers 1990;9(3):185–211.
19. What is Mindfulness? Mindful. Published July 8, 2020. Accessed August 25, 2023. https://www.mindful.org/what-is-mindfulness/.
20. Schuman-Olivier Z, Trombka M, Lovas DA, et al. Mindfulness and Behavior Change. Harv Rev Psychiatr 2020;28(6):371–94.
21. Ceravolo D, Raines DA. The Impact of a Mindfulness Intervention for Nurse Managers. J Holist Nurs 2019;37(1):47–55.
22. Paradiso L, Sweeney N. Just culture. Nurs Manag 2019;50(6):38–45.
23. Sachs CJ, Wheaton N. Second Victim Syndrome. In: StatPearls. StatPearls Publishing; 2023. Accessed August 25, 2023. http://www.ncbi.nlm.nih.gov/books/NBK572094/.
24. Truth and Reconciliation Commission of Canada. What We Have Learned: Principles of Truth and Reconciliation.; 194. www.trc.ca.

Cultural Humility and Diversity in Nursing Academia

Understanding History to Create a "Brave Space" Culture in the Classroom

Ashley Graham-Perel, EdD, RN, NPD-BC, MEDSURG-BC, CNE

KEYWORDS

• Diversity • Nursing education • Cultural humility • Nursing history

KEY POINTS

• Presentation of how to create a brave space in the classroom to foster cultural humility.
• Discussion of the importance of incorporating nursing history into academia.
• Describe the impact of diversity in nursing education and cultural humility.

INTRODUCTION

The teaching and integration of culture in nursing academia and practice have transcended with the profession's advancements over time. The tenet of culture is understood to be the ways of life, including beliefs and customs, among a group of people. Cultural humility, as discussed in this article, encompasses valuing differences among society with an awareness of the necessity to persistently learn, understand, and respect said differences.[1] The necessity to holistically meet the needs of patients, in the pursuit of health equity, mandates nursing academic leaders to appropriately prepare and support the next generation of nurses. However, in order to do so, historical progression in nursing academia and practice must first be introduced to students in the classroom. Nursing academicians are positioned at a critical juncture to mold the future generations of nursing with the skills of cultural humility, starting with fostering humility in the classroom. The dynamic culture of nursing education, with consideration of the diversity of nursing students and faculty, commands attention before the exploration of what is taught about the culture of patients. Classroom cultural humility must become the "brave space" of nursing academia. In this context, the concept of a "brave space" refers to the designing of an environment that welcomes

Columbia University School of Nursing, 560 West 168th Street, New York, NY 10032, USA
E-mail address: Ag4122@cumc.columbia.edu

Nurs Clin N Am 59 (2024) 11–19
https://doi.org/10.1016/j.cnur.2023.11.003
0029-6465/24/© 2023 Elsevier Inc. All rights reserved.

nursing.theclinics.com

all students and faculty to share in learning experiences that honors individual values while respecting the learning process. Key tenets of a brave space include "controversy with civility; owning intentions and impacts; challenge by choice; respect, and no attacks" (pp. 3–4).[2] This is possible with strategic approaches and revisiting the history of the culture of nursing education before trying to shape its future.

WHAT IS CULTURAL HUMILITY AND WHY IS DIVERSITY IMPORTANT?

Cultural humility is defined as, "having traits of respect, empathy, and critical self-reflection at both intrapersonal and interpersonal levels" (p. 278).[3] The nursing profession has transitioned over time from the practice of cultural competence to practicing cultural humility. Cultural competence in health care requires providers of care to recognize the cultural differences of their patients and gain knowledge about their respective cultural beliefs, practices, and lifestyle customs.[4] However, although these practices were a necessary foundation to develop an understanding of patient cultures, the foundation proved to be a fallacy because the health-care providers' general knowledge of cultures began to shift to detrimental stereotyping of patients.[5] In the article, "Rethinking Cultural Competence: Shifting to Cultural Humility," the authors stated,

> Culture is not stagnant, but a changing system of beliefs and values shaped by our interactions with one another, institutions, media, and technology, and by the socioeconomic determinants of our lives. Yet, the claim that one can become competent in any culture suggests that there is a core set of beliefs and values that remain unchanged and that are shared by all the members of a specific group. This static and totalizing view of culture that connotes a set of immutable ideas embraced by all members of a social group generates a social stereotype. (p.1)

The shift from cultural competence to cultural humility entails an adjustment in the approach to the culture of patients. Rather than the declaration of competence of another's culture, the practice of cultural humility is a consciousness of the limitations in fully understanding the expansive qualities of culture and proclaiming a commitment to continually learn about other cultures. Hughes and colleagues (2019)[1] described the realities of interpersonal and intrapersonal efforts required to fulfill cultural humility. They stated,

> The intrapersonal component involves an awareness of the limited ability to understand the worldview and culture of the patient. The interpersonal component incorporates a stance toward the patient that is marked by respect and an openness to the patient's worldview. (p.29)

A distinctive challenge of cultural humility in the classroom is linked to the lack of diversity noted in academia. This reality is then infiltrated from the classroom to the bedside. The deficiency of diversity among providers exacerbates the negative impact of cultural incompetence practices and furthers health-care disparities among patients.

Diversity of patient populations in relation to diversity of the nursing workforce remains an exigent impasse of cultural humility in health care that demands innovative approaches for resolutions. As the diversity of patient populations increases, researchers are looking into how nursing, as the largest health-care discipline, addresses the evolution of society's demographics. According to the American Association of Colleges of Nursing (2017)[6], the term diversity refers to the range of "individual, population, and social characteristics, including but not limited to age; sex;

race; ethnicity; sexual orientation; gender identity; family structures; geographic locations; national origin; immigrants and refugees; language; physical, functional and learning abilities; religious beliefs; and socioeconomic status." Evidence has demonstrated insufficiency in the percentages of diverse Registered Nurses and nursing students to adequately care for the ever-growing diverse population at hand.[7] Furthermore, research has linked the lack of diversity among health-care workers to health-care disparities and negative patient outcomes.[8] The consequences of a nursing workforce that lacks diversity furthers such deleterious outcomes due to unrecognized implicit biases; communication barriers between patients and providers; concerns of the lack of empathy; and mistrust from diverse patients.[9]

The transformation of the diversity of the United States population has been discussed at length in a myriad of research articles.[6,10,11] The United States Census Bureau has accentuated that although the current largest ethnic group in the nation is non-Hispanic Whites (at 58.9%),[12] this ethnic group is expected to decrease to 43.2% by the year 2060 (U.S. Census Bureau, 2015)[13]. By the year 2044, it is estimated that more than half of Americans, with a census increase to more than 400 million people, will belong to a minority group (any other group than non-Hispanic Whites alone). In fact, evidence proves that all other ethnic groups demonstrate an increase in percentages while the non-Hispanic Whites percentages persistently decrease.[13] The Census Bureau stated, "While all other groups experienced a natural increase (having more births than deaths) between 2015 and 2016, the non-Hispanic white alone group experienced a natural decrease of 163,300 nationally".[14] Continued discrepancies in nursing diversity will consequentially cause continued health-care disparities among underrepresented groups. This issue warrants an immediate action.

DIVERSITY IN NURSING EDUCATION

If one were to enter a nursing school and survey the demographics of the nurse educators in comparison with the demographics of the students, there would be a notable discrepancy in the findings. The American Association of Colleges of Nursing's (AACN) 2021 to 2022 report, *Enrollment and Graduations in Baccalaureate and Graduate Programs* in Nursing, presented that following statistics of enrollment of students from minority backgrounds in nursing programs: 40.8% of students in entry-level baccalaureate programs, 38.9% of master's students, 35.5% of students in research-focused doctoral programs, and 38.9% of Doctor of Nursing Practice (DNP) students.[9] The report also included statistics based on gender presenting the following data of male-identified enrolled students: 12.6% in baccalaureate programs, 11.7% in master's programs, 11.2% in research-focused doctoral studies, and 14.1% in DNP programs. The need to attract diverse nursing students is paralleled by the need to recruit more faculty from minority populations. The report concluded with the following statement, "Few nurses from racial/ethnic minority groups with advanced nursing degrees pursue faculty careers. According to 2021 data from AACN's annual survey, only 19.2% of full-time nursing school faculty come from minority backgrounds, and only 7.4% are male".[9]

Furthermore, if one were to study the diverse demographics of the nurse educators and link that data to the demographics of the patient populations, there would be nonequivalence of correlations among the findings. Deplorably, despite the growing diversity of the United States population, the nursing academic workforce has been regarded as an underrepresentation of the ethnicities at hand (AACN, 2023). Continued research is needed to identify the factors that have caused such depreciation. Research has found that the lack of minority nurse educators plays a role in the number of minority nursing students admitted to a university. The diversity of nursing students and patient populations is progressively cultivating; however, we cannot say the same for nurse educators in the academic setting. The AACN stated the following regarding this matter,

> A lack of minority nurse educators may send a signal to potential students that nursing does not value diversity or offer career ladder opportunities to advance through the profession. Students looking for academic role models to encourage and enrich their learning may be frustrated in their attempts to find mentors and a community of support. (p.3)

On conducting research on diversity in nursing academia, there is a notable deficiency in research addressing the lack of diversity among academic nursing faculty. The majority of the research conducted on diversity in nursing pertained to the diversity of the nursing students and hospital staff rather than the faculty[7,11,15]. However, as stated in the 2010 IOM report, a diverse student body will be able to relate to a diverse nursing faculty. If there is a continued shortage of diverse nursing educators, the challenges of attainment and retention of diverse nursing students will simultaneously persist.

HISTORY OF THE NURSING CULTURE (PRACTICE AND ACADEMIA)

As nursing academic leaders consider the ever-changing landscape of culture in society, it is germane to concurrently consider the history of the profession's academic culture. The history of nursing academia consists of a generally uniform faculty demographics identifying as White and female gendered. Structured along the helms of the late nineteenth century Florence Nightingale's school of nursing model, nursing academia is historically known to be strict, disciplined, and taxing with well-regarded expectations. Nightingale's standards also included a meticulous selection of young, esteemed White pupils to grow the nursing profession.[16] Tobell and D'Antonio (2022)[17] stated,

> Notions of class ran through these origin stories. Lest anyone miss the deeply held ideas about the importance of social hierarchies embedded in Nightingale's ideas about nursing, her notes Notes on Nursing for the Labouring Classes detailed the actual skills and techniques working-class women needed to show to their middle-class women employers who learned such supervisory skills from reading Notes on Nursing. These emerging leaders of nursing in the United States eschewed such obvious class distinctions. They, for example, never imported the two-tiered training model at St. Thomas', which had one program for "ladies" and another for those who needed to earn their living. Rather, the rhetoric stressed the need for the "right kind of woman" to enter nursing and enshrined the respectable middle-class virtues of honesty, faithfulness, truthfulness, obedience, and loyalty into the training of most other women who sought to become nurses. (p. 5)

The expectations of students, and faculty alike, ranged from one's duties, to your demeanor and representation as a nurse, to the quality of care and compassion elicited. For illustration, the following describes the culture of nursing education during the profession's steadfast increase from the 1900s to the 1920s. Deborah Judd (2010)[18] stated,

> As nurses' respectability increased, many still believed that the nurses of the day should only be associated with the emerging hospital systems and their judicious

control. Nurses' lives were influenced in essence by the hospital schools that accepted, trained, and eventually employed them; their duties and responsibilities were the direct result of the needs in these individual organizations at the end of the century. Nursing supervisors and physicians of the day determined their attire, the scope of their activities, and their schedules. (p. 67)

As nursing education advanced, the standardizations of nursing schools cultivated disputes of diversity and cultural humility. When considering the history of nursing education, one must reflect on who has historically been accepted as an educator or student in nursing. How has this shaped the culture of nursing education and what was the impact on those who did not meet the standards? Historical research of nursing education demonstrates that the educators and students of nursing were majorly of the white race. Due to segregation, especially but not exclusively in the southern states of the United States, diverse schools of nursing (based on race and gender) were established distinctly to meet the needs of diverse populations and provide access to education for those who were not accepted in general nursing programs.[19] One example that can be used is teaching about the establishment of diverse nursing schools throughout the country during segregation. For example, the Lincoln School for Nurses (LSN), 1898 to 1961 in the Bronx, New York, was established to educate Black women in the arts of nursing as admission of Black pupils was not granted in any other nursing school in the state.[20] The history of programs such as the LSN helps to develop trust with students as you discuss the history of nursing education and the recognition that nursing students were discriminated against, during admissions, and even beyond graduation. In addition, discrimination and biases were noted in the faculty at LSN because the faculties were predominantly of the white race, despite the institution being developed to educate a diverse group of students.

Presenting the history of nursing education to nursing students fosters discussions on the origins of nursing academia and some of the remnants that may still be felt today. Lewenson (2014)[21] presented examples of learning objectives and correlated them to historical moments in nursing history. There is much to be shared about the history of nursing and much more to be discovered. For instance, in the National Commission to Address Racism in Nursing's historical report series, nurse historians Dominique Tobell and Patricia D'Antonio (2022) stated the following,

We acknowledge the importance of topics and themes raised during the public comment period: the role of historically Black colleges and universities in nursing education and practice; the global histories of nursing, particularly those in Asia, the Middle East, and Africa; the experiences of Alaska Native nurses as well as Asian and Pacific Islander nurses in the U.S.; and the role of leadership and missions for nurses of color in those organizations that have emerged since the 1970s. Regrettably, these are topics for which richly contextualized historical studies do not yet exist. (p.4)

The current approaches to teaching cultural humility pose challenges for both nursing faculty and students. Students have reported, and demanded, that their faculty remain abreast of the latest cultural advancements of society and incorporate them into the curriculum accordingly.[22] Faculty have reported dedication to doing so; however, they also report anxiety about offending or misspeaking during lessons on cultures and sensitive matters.[23] The authors of the 2020 article, "Exploring Faculty Perceptions of Teaching Cultural Competence in Nursing" stated, "The universities and nursing programs should increase feelings of bravery and trust in the teaching environment and encourage faculty to create an open and comfortable multicultural classroom environment for learning, such as students feeling empowered to dialogue" (p.6). The impasse of student expectations and faculty efforts cultivates tense academic environments for both parties. In the 2010 article, "Cultural Diversity in Nursing Education: Perils, Pitfalls, and Pearls," the authors stated,

> Culture is acquired, dynamic, and largely unconscious. Culture is ubiquitous and often unexamined. Culture changes both through conscious effort, education, and experience, and by unplanned happenstance and history. Current American culture is concerned with the issue of political correctness, and the consequences for making an error in speech or action can be dramatic. Academic culture includes a raging debate about public and private speech, and many faculty members fear being labeled as insensitive or ignorant. It is much easier for individuals to teach what they were taught in the ways that they know than to venture out into the unfamiliar. (p.3)

The foundations of nursing education and its diversity have evolved. Consequently, the culture of nursing education continues to progress along with society. It is critical to acknowledge these changes and recognize that students, while committed to their education and the mission of health equity and social change, are entering nursing schools with high expectations of faculty. Students have voiced their desires for nursing curricula to parallel the diverse and steadfast changes in society.[24] Faculty is aware of the need to advance curriculum and lessons to meet societal needs and student requests. Nursing organizations have publicized their positionality on the importance of culturally competent nursing education and support for measures of innovations. The differentiating paradigms between the historical culture of nursing education and its current auspices are the relationships among faculty, students, and the academic institutions. We are no longer in the age of nursing education where the student experiences and education were completely determined by academic and hospital leaders. In terms of cultural humility, most practicing faculty may have been educated in such conditions, or similar conditions, and are putting forth the effort to deviate from their original culture of nursing education. There are cultural shifts between faculty and students. Having cultural humility in the classroom requires the acknowledgment of such shifts and strategies to not only respectfully mediate academic cultural differences but also establish common grounds on what the new "brave space" in the classroom looks like for all involved.

INCORPORATING CULTURAL HUMILITY IN ACADEMIA: MOVING FORWARD WHILE LOOKING BACK

When one walks into a classroom, the environment and subtleties of the relationships between faculty and students preserve deeply seeded historical truths of nursing education. Understanding nursing history promotes historical literacy and builds professional identity through historical exploration.[25] Matthias and Hundt (2023)[26] presented a roadmap for including history in the curriculum through adopting historical frameworks, using historical resources such as the American Association for the History of Nursing and historical databases, and publishing curriculum-based activities that integrate history to advance lesson plans.

Adapting to the diversity of the classroom is the responsibility of both faculty and students. In order to promote conversations on the culture of patients in health care, we must first cultivate a "brave space" climate for those in the classroom. Cultural humility in the classroom promotes respect and dignity for all participants. Smith and Foronda (2021)[27] recommend that faculty set ground rules at the beginning of the course and interactions with students. In their article, "Promoting Cultural Humility in

Nursing Education Through the Use of Ground Rules," the authors presented examples of ground rules in the table below. These ground rules include concepts of self-reflection, an open mind to continue learning, and respect toward the views and lifestyles of others.[27] Other strategies to incorporate cultural humility in academia include investigating the institution's culture and adjusting the mission and vision respectively to embrace cultural humility practices; training on cultural humility for all faculty and staff; and regularly assessing the evaluative standards for cultural humility (such as through student evaluations and institutional climate surveys; Hughes, and colleagues, 2019[1]; **Box 1**).

It is recommended by this author to preface these ground rules and strategies to incorporate cultural humility into academia with a discussion on the history of nursing education and the conditions of diversity within the classroom. The omission of history in nursing education deceives the student body's confidence in transparency. A few questions to discuss collectively are as follows: (1) What is my respective culture in terms of education? (2) What are the cultures of nursing education, historically? (3) What are the cultures of this academic institution? (4) Are there any areas of cultural shifts or shocks that may challenge teaching and learning? (5) What is my understanding of the culture of our classroom and how can I demonstrate efforts to learn new aspects of this culture? Discussion of these questions promotes cultural humility in the classroom and will build rapport between faculty and students. In order to learn how to best meet the cultural needs of patients, we must first consider how to best meet the needs of those in the classroom.

Cultural humility should be the "brave space" of the classroom, as we are all on the journey of learning and understanding the progressive nature of the nursing profession and the cultures of the communities we serve. As nursing education and its discipline

---

Box 1
Classroom ground rules based on cultural humility

1 I will enter each class with an open mind and possess an attitude willing to explore new concepts.

2 I will be aware of my personal values, beliefs, and behaviors and respect that others may not abide by the same values and belief system

3 I will focus on other's·feelings and experiences as well as my own.

4 I will enter each class with a flexible and humble attitude and not allow my ego to impede the learning experience.

5 I will engage in healthy, supportive interactions with my professor and peers to help foster an engaging learning environment.

6 I will engage in self-reflections as a lifelong learner and strive to critique my thoughts, actions, and behaviors as I interact with people who have both similar and opposing views as myself.

7 I will attempt to embrace conflicting viewpoints by giving them my full consideration.

8 I will support my peers as we engage in discussions and learning.

9 I will try to recognize power difference and minimize them.

10 I will strive to demonstrate respect for my professor and my peers.

Reprinted from Smith, A.; Foronda, C. (2021). Promoting Cultural Humility in Nursing Education Through the Use of Ground Rules. Nursing Education Perspectives, 42,[2] 117 to 119.

advances, valuing of the multifaceted, cultural dimensions of education from the perspectives of faculty and students is critical. Acknowledgments of the varied experiences and expectations of nursing education, coupled with the professional legacy we all inherit as Registered Nurses, should serve as a grounding tenet of classroom cultural humility. The inclusion of nursing history is the catalyst for this journey, elucidating the impact of the past while forging a path for the future.

CLINICS CARE POINTS

- The consequences of a nursing workforce that lacks diversity furthers the deleterious outcomes of health disparities due to unrecognized implicit biases; communication barriers between patients and providers; concerns of the lack of empathy, and mistrust from diverse patients.
- As nursing education and its discipline advances, valuing of the multifaceted, cultural dimensions of edcuation from perspectives of faculty and students is critical.
- Nursing students have reported, and demanded, that their faculty remain abreast of the latest cultural advancements of society and incorporate them into the curriculum accordingly.
- Incorporation of nursing history in academia bridges the gap of cultural humility in nursing practice.

DISCLOSURE

The author declares no potential conflicts of interest with respect to research, authorship, and/or publication of this article.

REFERENCES

1. Hughes V, Delva S, Nkimbeng M, et al. Not missing the opportunity: Strategies to promote cultural humility among future nursing faculty. J Prof Nurs 2019;36: 28–33.
2. Ali D. Safe spaces and brave spaces historical context and Recommendations for student Affairs professionals. NASPA: Research and Policy Institute; 2017. p. 1–13.
3. Hook JN. Engaging Patients with Cultural Humility. J Psychol Christianity 2014;277–80.
4. Lekas HM, Pahl K, Lewis C. Rethinking Cultural Competence: Shifting to Cultural Humility. Health Services Insight 2020;13:1–4.
5. Dreher M, MacNaughton N. Cultural competence in nursing: Foundation or Fallacy? Nurs Outlook 2002;181–6.
6. American Association of Colleges of Nursing (AACN). (2017, March 20). American Association of Colleges of Nursing. Retrieved from Diversity, Inclusion, & Equity in Academic Nursing: AACN Position Statement: https://www.aacnnursing. org/Portals/42/Diversity/AACN-Position-Statement-Diversity-Inclusion.pdf.
7. Phillips J, Malone B. Jan-Feb). Increasing Racial/Ethnic Diversity in Nursing to Reduce Health Disparities and Achieve Health Equity. Publich Health Reports 2014;129(2):45–50.
8. Travers J, Smaldone A, Cohn E. Does State Legislation Improve Nursing Workforce Diversity? Policy Polit Nurs Pract 2015;16:109–16.

9. AACN. (2023, April 10). Enhancing Diversity in the Nursing Workforce. Retrieved from American Association of Colleges of Nursing: https://www.aacnnursing.org/News-Information/Fact-Sheets/Enhancing-Diversity.

10. Koch J, Everett B, Phillips J, et al. Diversity characteristics and the experiences of nursing students during clinical placements: A qualitative study of student, faculty and supervisors' views. Contemp Nurse 2014;15–25.

11. LaVeist T. Integrating the 3Ds-Social Determinants, Health Disparities, and Health-Care Workforce Diversity. Publich Health Records 2014;9–14.

12. U.S. Census Bureau. (2023, August 10). United States Census Bureau. Retrieved from U.S. Census Bureau Quick Facts: https://www.census.gov/quickfacts/fact/table/US/PST045222.

13. U.S. Census Bureau. (2015, March). Projections of the Size and Composition of the U.S. Population: 2014 to 2060: Population Estimates and Projections. Retrieved February 20, 2019, from The United States Census Bureau: https://www.census.gov/content/dam/Census/library/publications/2015/demo/p25-1143.pdf.

14. U.S. Census Bureau. (2017, June 22). The Nation's Older Population Is Still Growing, Census Bureau Reports. Retrieved April 3, 2019, from The U.S. Census Bureau: https://www.census.gov/newsroom/press-releases/2017/cb17-100.html.

15. Tabi M, Thornton K, Gaino M, et al. Minority Nursing Students' Perception of Their Baccalaureate Program. J Nurs Educ Pract 2013;3(9):167–75.

16. Hine D. Black women in white: racial conflict and cooperation in the nursing profession 1890-1950. Bloomington & Indianapolis: Indiana University Press; 1989.

17. Tobbell D, D'Antonio P. The history of racism in nursing: a review of existing scholarship. National Commission to Address Racism in Nursing; 2022.

18. Judd D. A New Century Brings Novel Ideas and Social Concerns. In: Judd D, Sitzman K, Davis M, editors. A history of American nursing: trends and eras. Sudbury: Jones and Bartlett Publishers; 2010. p. 60–93.

19. Ervin S. Chapter 1: History of Nursing Education in the United States. In: Keating S, DeBoor S, editors. Curriculum Development and evaluation in nursing education. 4th Edition. New York: Springer Publishing Company; 2017. p. 5–26.

20. Graham-Perel, A. (2021) Color Me Capable: the Rise of African American nurse Faculty at Lincoln School for nurses, 1898 to 1961 (doctoral Dissertation, Teachers College Columbia University) Columbia Academic Commons. Available at: https://doi.org/10.7916/d8-yz46-f337.

21. Lewenson S. Integrating Nursing History into the Curriculum. J Prof Nurs 2004;20(6):374–80.

22. Anton-Solanas I, Tambo-Lizalde E, Haman-Alcober N, et al. Nursing Students' Experience of Learning Cultural Competence. PLoS One 2021;1–24.

23. Chen H, Jensen F, Chung J, et al. Exploring faculty perceptions of teaching cultural competence in nursing. Teach Learn Nurs 2020;15(1):1–6.

24. Bednarz H, Schim S, Doorenbos A. Cultural Diversity in Nursing Education: Perils, Pitfalls, and Pearls. J Nurs Educ 2010;49(5):253–60.

25. Smith K, Brown A, Crookes P. History as reflective practice: A model for integrating historical studies into nurse education. Collegian 2014;22(3):341–7.

26. Matthias A, Hundt B. The Power of the Past: A Roadmap for Integrating Nursing History into the Curriculum. J Prof Nurs 2023;46:231–7.

27. Smith A, Foronda C. Promoting Cultural Humility in Nursing Education Through the Use of Ground Rules. Nurs Educ Perspect 2021;42(2):117–9.

Meeting the Religious and Cultural Needs of Patients at Different Points in Their Care

Check for updates

Terry Throckmorton, PhD, RN[a],
Lucindra Campbell-Law, PhD, APRN, ANP, PMHNP-BC[a],*

KEYWORDS

- Holistic care • Culture • Religion

KEY POINTS

- True holistic care implies an in-depth assessment and understanding of patient needs based on their physical, social, psychological, and spiritual makeup.
- Understanding the beliefs and cultural influences that contribute to patient decisions should provide some insights into the appropriate approach to these patients and the best ways to incorporate positive health-care practices into their lives.
- A common insight to each group is respect, a gentle greeting as a handshake, and a discreet approach to assessing their practices and needs.

MEETING THE RELIGIOUS AND CULTURAL NEEDS OF PATIENTS AT DIFFERENT POINTS IN THEIR CARE

True holistic care implies an in-depth assessment and understanding of each patient's needs based on their physical, social, psychological, and spiritual makeup.[1] These parameters are affected by their native culture as well as their adopted culture. A patient's culture is composed of beliefs, values, and lifestyles to successfully manage life changes and development.[2] Understanding the general elements of specific cultures and religions can provide a basis for more insightful inquiry with patients regarding their preferences in health care. Because religion and culture are often intertwined, a focus on these 2 influences on patient perspectives is an inherent factor in the provision of care for the whole person.

In the United States and in many other countries, much of the population is integrated with people from a variety of cultures and religions. Approaching patients based purely on their apparent ethnicity and assumed related religion is often a mistake. In the past, most countries had a dominant ethnic group and a dominant

[a] University of St. Thomas, Peavy School of Nursing, 3800 Montrose Boulevard, Houston, TX 77006, USA
* Corresponding author. PO Box 1188, Stafford, TX 77497.
E-mail address: campbell@stthom.edu

Nurs Clin N Am 59 (2024) 21–35
https://doi.org/10.1016/j.cnur.2023.11.004
0029-6465/24/© 2023 Elsevier Inc. All rights reserved.

nursing.theclinics.com

religion or group of related religions such as Islamic or Christian but because of missionary work across the world, many ethnic groups have members who espouse different religions or have no religious affiliation. Those with no religious affiliation may or may not believe in a God. Approximately 16% of the world population is not affiliated with a religion.[3]

For nurses working at the bedside, identifying cultural and religious preferences of a patient may be difficult. Approaching patients of different ethnicities and potential religious beliefs other than their own may be even more difficult. Most clinicians are comfortable with their own religious beliefs but experience discomfort or uncertainty when approaching a patient with different beliefs[4,5] and few address spiritual/religious issues with the patient. Barriers to addressing spiritual/cultural concerns have been listed as time, lack of knowledge of resources, and the opinion that these concerns were better addressed by chaplains. Choi and colleagues (2019)[5] found that although more nurses than attending physicians or fellows addressed these issues with patients, the number was still only about 26% of those surveyed.

Considering the complexities of addressing spiritual and cultural needs of patients, the preparation of most nurses and interdisciplinary staff is limited. Recommendations for increased education for all health-care providers have been suggested.[6] In addition to formal education, practical guides for clinicians that outline basic beliefs and practices for various religions and ethnicities can be helpful. This article includes basic beliefs and practices related to Native Americans and Alaska Natives (NA/ANs), Jewish people (ethno-religious group), Filipinos, Islamic people (Muslims), and Hispanic/Latino American people. Points in care addressed in this article include birth, general health-care considerations, and death. General beliefs are presented as a baseline to better understand each patient's perspective.

NATIVE AMERICANS AND ALASKA NATIVES
General Considerations

By 2013, there were approximately 6.5 million NA/ANs in the 574 federally recognized tribes in the United States.[7] Although many Native Americans live in tribal nations and villages and are cared for by the Indian Health Services, Native Americans are often treated in hospitals located near reservations. Understanding the general history of health care and personal beliefs about pregnancy, medical care, and death is a basis for providing holistic care for this group of patients.

The beliefs and languages of NA/ANs are as varied as the tribal entities.[8] There are some commonalities that can be used in planning care. A basic tenet of NA/AN life is the belief that all persons, places, and things have a role in maintaining harmony and balance. NA/AN traditions center around events in the life cycle including birth, achievement of adulthood, marriage, and death. NA/ANs expect dignity, honesty, and compassion in their interactions and as with many tribes and other cultures value listening, mutual respect, dignity, and harmony in their daily activities.[9] They expect professional behavior from health-care givers but also respect humor in communication. NA/ANs value family and extended family and recognize shared responsibilities.

The term American Indian or Native American refers to individuals living in the 49 lower states and Alaska Natives to those who reside in Alaska.[9] These titles reflect an indigenous status. According to the United Nations (6006),[10] indigenous people identify themselves as native to an area and are accepted by the community as such. They have an in-depth connection to specific territories and natural resources, have developed distinct social, economic, and political systems in addition to their own language, beliefs, and culture. NA/ANs live in many large cities as well as rural areas and tribal communities. It is not uncommon for NA/AN people to speak English, plus one or more other languages such as Spanish or French. Many NA/ANs exist in a dual world, incorporating both traditional and contemporary values. Values are first derived from family, then clan, and tribe.

As with many cultures, gender differences and roles are defined and the roles may vary with marriage. Unwritten rules may govern communications among men, women, and between men and women including those related to touching and eye contact. These rules may not be evident, and understanding may need to rely on observation of body language. When possible, same-gender caregivers should be assigned to NA/AN patients, and their modesty respected.[11] Women may refer to their menstrual period as moon time and consider that time one of power.

Specific procedures such as x-rays or MRIs may be considered in the same manner as photographs. A detailed explanation and request for permission should be provided. Surgery that includes the removal of body parts should also be carefully explained. Because traditions regarding body parts may vary among different tribes, the patients should be asked about their preference for disposition of the body part.[11] Patients may be reluctant to express pain or other symptoms because these symptoms may indicate that their bodies are failing them. Researchers have determined that NA and ANs, especially younger men with less education and a high perception of pain may tend to use alcohol, marijuana, or other illegal drugs to manage pain.[12] Other patients may decline pain medication for fear of becoming addicted.[11]

Authority is conferred with age and to persons in positions of authority.[11] A drawback of considering physicians and nurses as persons with authority is that they may just communicate what they think the health-care provider wants to hear. In greeting new patients, a gentle handshake is considered a sign of respect. A period of silence after the greeting may occur and should not be interrupted. Direct eye contact may be avoided in respect of an authority figure. Listening is very important. Silence usually indicates that the person is thinking about what has been said. Direct questions are not always acceptable. Indirect approaches to obtaining information are usually more acceptable. Body language is important and may indicate that the patient is uncomfortable. Criticism of others is also unacceptable. Scheduling appointments requires a detailed approach with more than one method of reminder because the recognition of calendar and clock time may vary.

Health, for the individual Native American and Alaska Native, is based on appropriate interactions with the spiritual world.[13] Well-being is based on synchrony with the forces of Nature and the universe. Illness is a sign that the person is out of step with these forces causing a lack of harmony within the spirit, mind, and body.[13] Health-care practices may include a combination of holistic and allopathic care.[14] The patients may therefore request that the elder or medicine man be permitted to treat them as well as a health-care professional and may also ask to incorporate other complementary therapies.

Spirituality is usually community-based and is integral to life. It is expressed in ceremonies, religious events, and practices. Tribal elders are often the recognized religious authorities. Just as with chaplains and representatives of other religions, these religious leaders should have access to the patient when requested. Respect can be communicated to the patient and Tribal elder by not touching religious icons and avoiding intrusive questions about the religious practices.

Childbirth

Traditionally, Native American, and Alaska Native women took special care of themselves during pregnancy.[15] They not only avoided foods and activities that they thought could be harmful to the pregnancy but also cared for their minds and spirits.[16] Pregnant women sought to maintain a sense of peace, avoiding negative thoughts and arguments. As with many other indigenous people, birth may be viewed as a ritual to celebrate new life. The child passes from a spiritual existence to a physical life. Traditional women may have asked a medicine man to ensure a positive delivery. The expectant parents may have also engaged in rituals such as daily hand washing.

Modern NA and AN women may not practice traditional activities but may continue to focus on a healthy pregnancy. Many modern NA/AN women still prefer the upright position for delivery.[17] Many may also want to hasten the delivery and may use herbal substances for that purpose. They may use herbs and teas during labor for other purposes, sing a special song, and request the presence of a midwife, family members, and spiritual leaders.[11] Women may request that the placenta be saved. Circumcision of male infants is not usually done. The sanctity of life is highly valued but abortion practices may vary. Nurses can facilitate the best mingling of pregnancy and delivery practices by supporting those that pose no harm to the baby such as the upright position for delivery and explaining the potential harm of some herbs and other products.

Cultural practices around birth may include ceremonies for welcoming and celebrating the new life and the sharing of traditional knowledge and teachings with the infant to welcome the child into the community.[18] Ceremonies implemented at birth may include stories relating to a connection to the land.[16] These practices are all positive and should be incorporated into the care of the newborn infant when requested. When ceremonies or rituals are performed, caregivers may be expected to leave the room.

Death

The practices around death, such as those around birth, vary according to the tribe. Death rituals may include face painting, feathers tied around the head as a prayer, and dressing the patient in traditional clothing.[7] Death is considered a natural part of life but the approach to death depends on whether the patient fears or accepts death.[7] Native Americans use food to honor the dying and deceased as opposed to flowers.[11] Patients may request a religious representative based on their specific beliefs.

The body of the patient is considered sacred by most tribes but customs related to burial and any memorial rituals vary by tribe and location.[7] The body should not be moved until the family has specified their desired practices.[11] The family may request that the patient be covered by a blanket at the time of death. Selected ceremonial objects may be placed with the body. The family may cut a lock of hair from the deceased person, especially if the patient is a child. Traditional NA/ANs do not generally approve of embalming. They may request to stay with the body for long periods. This time can extend for as long as 4 days. It is very important to the family that the caregiver learns their preferences before any actions related to their deceased family member.

JEWISH CULTURE AND RELIGION (ETHNO-RELIGIOUS GROUP)
General Considerations

In 2021, the Pew Research Center estimated that approximately 5.8 million adults in the United States identified as Jewish including 4.2 million who specified practicing the Jewish religion and 1.5 million who identified as Jewish but with no religion.[19] They found that approximately 1.8 million children were being raised in the Jewish religion. Jewish American adults generally identify as non-Hispanic White but approximately 8% identify with other races. At least 17% of American Jews live in multiracial homes.[20] As the US population has increased, the Jewish population has proportionately increased. Most nurses will encounter Jewish patients in their area of practice at some time in their careers.

There are 3 primary Jewish denominations or streams among American Jews. The denominations differ from one another based on their application of Jewish tradition, and their interpretation and fidelity to traditional Jewish law.[21] They include Reform, Conservative, and Orthodox Judaism. Reform Judaism focuses on tradition over Jewish law, seeks to adjust tradition to modern interpretation, and places emphasis on personal choice for observing rituals. Conservative Judaism occupies a central point regarding Orthodox and Reform Judaism, adopting some concessions to modern life but maintaining some traditions such as keeping kosher and avoiding intermarriage. Orthodox Judaism prescribes adherence to the traditional understanding of Jewish law. These laws include adherence to Shabbat with no driving, turning electricity on and off, or handling money and remaining kosher.

Basic tenets of the Jewish faith include loving your neighbor as yourself and that all humans are created in the image of God, meaning that every human life has value that is immeasurable, is equal, and is unique.[22] These tenets imply that providers will approach patients with respect and carefully ask questions related to the plan of care.[23] Jewish holidays include Passover (the most celebrated), Shavuot, Rosh Hashanah, and Yom Kippur (considered High Holy Days), Sukkot, and Chanukah. Patients hospitalized in Yom Kippur may want to fast and deny various luxuries for themselves. Jewish patients may want to pray 3 times a day, in the morning, afternoon, and evening. In addition, each time they eat or drink they say a blessing before and afterward.

Jewish patients who remain kosher can usually obtain prepackaged foods from food services in most hospitals.[24] If the patient's care requires food that is not on the kosher diet, the food may be given if the patient's life is in jeopardy. Often, a kosher alternative can be found. Most medications are acceptable; however, chewable and milky preparations may be problematic. It is always appropriate to check with the person's Rabbi. During Passover, leavened bread and other foods are forbidden. During this time, patients may require that all their food be kosher.

Some Jewish men and women wear head coverings. Some grow beards and have special sidelocks.[24] Observant Jews wash their hands 3 times using a cup and wash their hands before a meal in which bread is eaten. Boys begin observant practices at age 13 and girls at 12 years of age; however, children should not be given nonkosher meals without parental consent. When caring for Jewish patients, their modesty is important and should always be honored.

Most forms of treatment are allowable under the mandate that the saving of a life is paramount.[24] When treatment is critical to continued life, all medical treatments should be implemented. Jewish law does not include specific guidelines for abortion, organ transplant or donation, life-threatening treatments, removal of life support, genetic-based treatment, infertility treatment, or contraception. The patient may want to consult a Rabbi.

Childbirth

Jewish law indicates that life begins at birth.[24] Some parents do not allow baby showers or plan for the child until the child is born. A Cesarean section is permitted and almost any procedure is permitted to save the mother's or baby's life. Jewish women refrain from sexual relations for 7 days after the birth of a boy and for 14 days after the birth of a girl.

Brit Milah or circumcision is one of the most observed Jewish rituals. It is performed on males on the eighth day after birth during the day and is called a bris. A sandak, usually a grandparent or a rabbi, holds the child, and a mohel performs the circumcision.[25] It is important to ascertain from the parents if they choose to have their son circumcised in the Jewish tradition on the eighth day rather than in the hospital.

Death

Jewish people believe that death is part of the natural process and that there is an afterlife where each person is rewarded.[26] Jewish law does allow caregivers to remove a person from prolongation of life on a ventilator when death is pending, and the person is suffering. After a person dies, their eyes are closed, and they are placed on the floor. In the hospital, they will remain in bed. The body is never left alone, and there is no food or drink consumed in the room with the person. The body is washed and clothed in a linen shroud. Autopsies are discouraged and if mandated should be minimally invasive. The body is not embalmed, and cremation is not permitted. The body should be released to the family as soon as possible.

There are many mourning rituals and specifications for the burial and the gravesite. For caregivers, it is important to realize that there are mourning rituals and that many people may be involved. Rituals in the hospital are relatively simple and are supported by most health-care institutions.

FILIPINOS

At the heart of the Filipino culture is "kapwa" indicating that persons who are treated as "kapwa" have a shared inner strength and can identify with the other person.[27] Filipinos focus on their families, celebrations, and other festivities. Because of the many difficulties in their native country, they may have a philosophy of accepting whatever happens. Their coping practices may include patience, flexibility, humor, and fatalistic resignation. When ill, they may also feel shame and sensitivity to criticism.

Spirituality is a strong feature of the culture. Religion is an ever-present influence, and many Filipinos are Catholic. Hospitality is a strong feature of any interface with Filipinos including an abundant offering of food. Filipinos are industrious, generous, and have great respect for their elders. Staring or looking directly at people with whom they are talking is usually seen as impolite.[28] This should not be viewed as mistrust or lack of confidence. Tagalog (Filipino) is the national language but English is also common. Filipinos also speak several other languages; the most common are Ilocano and Visayan.

Many Filipino Americans migrated to the United States years ago and have adopted American health-care practices.[29] Those who have arrived more recently may tend to adhere to traditional indigenous healing practices. Those who originated from rural areas and emigrated later in life may still rely on indigenous healing practices and may wait until late to seek help. Filipinos rely on family and friends for support in illness.

Childbirth

Filipino women focus on healthy behaviors and avoiding certain practices such as wearing nail polish and cutting their hair during pregnancy.[30] It is common for relatives to visit; however, some mothers will not want visitors to stand in or near the door or touch the mother because the mother may fear that difficulties with labor will occur. In the Philippines, burying the placenta is a tradition as a conclusion to labor pain and the beginning of womb healing.

Death

Death in the family is an important event and is viewed as an opportunity to enhance family ties.[31] Family members and friends will mourn the deceased member but a happy atmosphere is supported to send the person on the journey to the afterlife. Several rituals surround the death including the "Siyam Na Araw," which is a 9-day novena with prayers and masses for the deceased. A 40-day mourning period follows death ending with a ceremonial mass. This practice is based on the belief that Christ rose to heaven after 40 days.

ISLAMIC PEOPLE (MUSLIMS)

Muslims represent approximately 25% of the world's population.[32] There are an estimated 1.8 billion followers. People who follow the Islamic religion are called Muslims. Followers believe in one true God, Allah. The 2 primary sects within the Muslim religion are the Sunnis and the Shiites with most Muslims being Sunni. Muslims are expected to pray 5 times each day with a prayer ritual.[33] The prayer space should be quiet and free of human images. Muslims are expected to wash before prayer. Patients may need assistance with the ablutions. Muslim women may wear a hijab to cover their hair or niquab or burka, which covers much of the body. The holy book of the Muslim religion is the Quran. Muslims fast and refrain from alcohol, smoking, and sex from dawn to sunset.

Muslims view illness as a test from God and approach it with prayers.[33] Maintaining a healthy body is considered a duty. They view providing care for people who are ill as a responsibility of society. Exemptions from fasting include children before puberty, elderly who cannot fast, nursing mothers, pregnant women, those who are menstruating, and those who are ill. People who are ill can make up fasting later. During Ramadan, emergency treatment can be given. Nonemergency treatments can be given after sunset when possible. Blood transfusions are permitted but patients may prefer donations from individuals they know.[33] Muslims in general may use temporary contraceptive methods. Vasectomy and tubal ligation are permitted if additional pregnancies threaten the woman's health. Abortion is not permitted after 120 days.[34] They would want the fetus to receive a proper burial.[33]

The Muslim diet excludes alcohol and pork.[34] They follow halal preparation of meats and poultry. There are certified Muslim food distributors that can provide food to hospitals. When this is not possible, acceptable foods such as vegetables, eggs, milk, and fish can be served. Medications with pork extract coatings and those containing alcohol should be avoided.

Muslim men and women maintain modest dress and often cover their heads.[33,35] Women may wish to wear the head covering in the hospital or will ask that individuals knock before entering so that the covering can be replaced. Every effort should be made to respect the patient's privacy. Muslims may not choose to shake hands with members of the opposite sex and may request a same-sex caregiver.

Childbirth

Muslims generally will accept assisted reproductive technologies; however, donor sperm use, and cryopreserved sperm when the father has expired, and surrogacy are not permitted.[34] Before conception, Muslims believe that the child has the right to birth within a legal union, with the ability to know its parents.[35] They believe that the child has the right to an acceptable name, to be nursed, educated, and to be raised in a loving situation.

Soon after birth, the father or respected member of the community whispers the name of Allah followed by the declaration of Faith. This rite is usually performed in privacy.[32,35] Soon after, before the infant begins feedings, a small piece of date is rubbed on the roof of the infant's mouth by a respected person to transmit positive attributes.

A third ritual is the tying of a small pouch containing a prayer around the infant's wrist or neck to protect the baby from harm. Circumcision is required of male babies and preferably occurs within the first 7 days of life. If there are medical concerns, it can be performed during later childhood years.

Death

Because Muslims believe in predestination by God, they are often fairly accepting of death.[34] Treatment of patients to prolong life is not required in the final period of life. Islam views life as sacred and therefore suicide and euthanasia are forbidden. It is essential that family members be notified when a patient is dying. Many families will want to be present to pray with the patient. In the absence of the family, the imam on-call can counsel the patient.

After death, family or community members wash the body of the dead and bury the person as quickly as possible. Cremation is not allowed, and embalming is not performed unless required by law. The imam on-call or the local mosque must be notified immediately to accommodate Janaza (funeral) service.[32] Usually, the family will grieve with others for a maximum of 3 days and then grieve in private.[34]

HISPANIC/LATINO AMERICAN PEOPLE

Hispanic/Latino/Latinx people represented 19.1% of the United States population by 2022 with 333,287,557 people.[36] This estimate represents an increase from 2020 of 0.6%. The US government classifies Hispanic Latino Americans as immigrants or natural citizens tracing their roots to Spain, Mexico, Central America, South America, and the Spanish-speaking nations of the Caribbean. Each of these entities has its own dialect, beliefs, and folklore as well as differences among individuals living in rural and urban areas.

An interesting finding of the 2022 census was that 75.5% considered themselves as White, whereas 21.5% considered themselves to be Black/African American, American Indian/Alaska Native, Asian, or Native Hawaiian/Pacific Islander, and 3% considered themselves to be of more than one race. Only 14.6% were foreign-born. Of those reporting, 88.9% of those aged 25 years or older had a high school education or higher and 33.7% of those aged 25 years or older had a bachelor's degree or higher. Those aged younger than 65 years who reported a disability represented 8.7% and those aged younger than 65 years without health insurance included 0.3%.

Hispanic patients and parents seen in health-care institutions may speak only Spanish, both English and Spanish, or other languages, or English only. In a single-site study of Hispanic parents, Fowler and colleagues (2022)[37] found that 77% of the respondents spoke only Spanish. It is important to determine immediately whether an interpreter is needed and whether the interpreter understands specific Spanish dialects. However, the Pew Research Center (2023)[38] in their 2022 survey found a significant increase in the number of Hispanics who spoke English. This change from previous years is partially due to the decrease in the percentage (32%) of all US Hispanics who were immigrants with US births to Hispanic parents at a higher percentage than the arrival of new immigrants in 2022. Depending on the location in the United States, the language spoken by patients may or may not be English.

Hispanic beliefs may vary according to whether they emigrated to the United States or were born in the country. For the Hispanic population, family is the center of support for education, enculturation, socialization, and is a safety net for family members.[39] Because the family is often multigenerational, each patient has a strong cadre of supporters during illness. For the health-care provider, this fact can be either a strength or a deficit depending on how well the caregiver relates to the family.

Hispanic families usually have well-defined roles for the father, the wage earner, and the mother, the homemaker. These gender role depictions in Hispanic cultures are indicated as machismo and marianismo.[39] Machismo, in the past, has been described as hypermasculinity. It has sometimes been associated with spouse abuse. A newer, more positive male role characterization (caballerismo) is being seen including characteristics such as chivalry, bravery, and family provider attributes. The caballerismo role behaviors have been associated with better health promotion practices.[39,40] Marianista expectations that the wife or mother be the primary source of strength and manage the family's overall well-being and spiritual growth may lead to psychological burdens for women.

Families often perpetuate the belief in folk illnesses and folk medicines for family members. Understanding the basic concepts of folk illnesses and their treatments and how they relate to traditional American medicine provides a strong basis for managing illness in this population. Fowler and colleagues (2022)[37] found that 85% of 200 Hispanic parents indicated a belief in one or more folk illnesses. The most common illnesses included colico (colic related to coldness in the stomach), empacho (gastrointestinal obstruction), and mal de ojo (a hex placed on children by a powerful person). Belief in folk illnesses was more common in parents born outside the United States. There are many folk illnesses, and it is important to determine if the patient believes in specific illnesses and how they relate to traditionally defined illnesses. Respect for patient beliefs will provide a basis for positive outcomes.

Folk remedies commonly used include bathing (banos), herbs in the form of teas, massage, oils, and ointments.[37] Many patients who have used folk remedies or would like to use them do not discuss them with their caregivers. Keeping an open mind to alternative/complementary approaches can facilitate more open communication. Often the folk treatment causes no harm and may add to improvement.

Childbirth

For many Hispanic women, adherence to folk practices may inhibit their participation in preventive health care including prenatal care. If they are living in traditionally paternalistic families, they may hesitate to take charge of their own health care. However, historically, Hispanic women have taken good care of themselves during pregnancy. An occurrence termed the Latina Health Paradox refers to the favorable birth outcomes equal to or better than national averages in the United States.[40,41] Researchers have attributed this result to beliefs about pregnancy and motherhood and the pregnant woman's healthy behavior before and during pregnancy. Hispanic women believe that pregnancy is a normal event in life. This belief may result in a later initiation of prenatal care.

Pregnant women may avoid certain foods, events such as funerals, and intercourse for fear of harming the baby.[40] Picas may be experienced by Hispanic women, and they may not realize that the cravings and ingestions should be reported. Some believe that drinking milk and taking vitamins such as those with folic acid cause weight gain and larger babies and avoid it. Patients may drink chamomile tea to ease labor, ruda con chocolate (common/garden rue with chocolate)[42] to speed labor, and a Mexican herb, epazote, to clean the stomach after delivery. Asking about diet is important.

Hispanics patients may fear epidurals and anesthesia as potentially life threatening.[40] They may prefer natural delivery without medications. After delivery, Hispanic women may observe cuarentena, a 40-day recuperation period after childbirth.[43] They may avoid showers for a few days, avoid heavy lifting, and hot meals and receive support from family and friends. Because some may not want to leave home for a period after birth, they may miss the first postpartum visit.

Breastfeeding among Hispanic women is both a cultural and familial expectation.[44] Hispanic women say they would prefer to breastfeed because they know the benefits for child and mother but feel embarrassed doing so in the United States. In addition, many women experience pressure to work. Providing additional support for breastfeeding among Hispanic may be important to their success.

Practices surrounding the infant may include avoidance of the "mal de ojo" (evil eye), placement of a worry doll in the bed, lighting candles with or without prayers, swaddling the baby with the legs straight, and the use of Vicks VapoRub (Vivaporu) for most ailments.[45] Bracelets are placed on the arm of the infant to ward off evil eye and visitors admiring the baby are encouraged to touch the infant. Worry dolls are placed in the bed so that the child can discuss their worries with the doll. Velitas or candles are used whenever the mother would like something for her baby or when the child is ill. Tightly swaddling the infant with the legs straight is thought to prevent bowing of the legs; however, forcing the legs is contraindicated to prevent damage to soft cartilage and hip dysplasia. Some mothers use Vicks as a cure all and apply it to the chest and sometimes the feet. Mothers may also avoid cutting the baby's hair until the baby is 1 year old thinking that cutting it may affect the quality and growth of hair later in life. Although many of these practices are harmless, it is important to inquire about any practices that are not prescribed by the health-care team.

Death

For Hispanics, dying is considered as part of the life cycle, and the dead usually are fondly remembered.[46] Discussions related to death and palliative care may be avoided and the family may request that the discussion occur between the family and the patient. The family may feel that talking about death may hasten the death of their loved one. When patients die in the hospital, there may be a fear that the deceased person may become confused and have difficulty finding the way to the afterlife. Consistent with folklore and the influence of the Catholic Church, the family may place rosary beads and prayer cards with the patient. The prayer cards usually contain a picture of a saint, Christ, or the blessed virgin and a prayer for the dying person. In the home, votive candles will also be placed at the bedside.

In the Hispanic culture, caring for the sick and the dying is the responsibility of women.[46] For those who adhere to Catholicism, both anointing of the sick and last rites (Extreme Unction) will be performed. The anointing of the sick is a blessing by a priest, and the last rites involve a blessing and final confession. Allowing privacy for these sacraments will be important for the patient and family. The family may wish to bathe the patient after death. The mourning process may be long with a large wake and mass and therefore embalming is common. Cremation is often allowed but many choose burial according to Catholic beliefs. Organ donation is viewed with some skepticism, and the donation rate is generally low.[47,48]

SUMMARY

This article was written to provide basic background information for 5 patient populations: NA/ANs (indigenous populations), Jewish people (ethno-religious group), Filipinos, Islamic people (Muslims), and Hispanic/Latino/Latinx Americans. Understanding the beliefs and cultural influences that contribute to patient decisions should provide some insights into the appropriate approach to these patients and the best ways to incorporate positive health-care practices into their lives. Although each culture or religion has specific practices attributed to it, people who espouse these cultures and religions may not practice the tenets to the same degree. Individuals interpret their cultural and religious practices within unique frameworks often developed according to family or peer practices.

Multiple terms and competencies have been proposed during the last 10 years related to the care of individuals from different cultures, including cultural awareness, cultural sensitivity, cultural competence, cultural humility, and cultural responsiveness. Perhaps, the most important of these concepts for holistic care are awareness that individuals are different from each other both within and between cultures or religions and that caregivers are not experts in patient cultures and perspectives but learners (cultural humility).

Patient-centered care requires that the caregiver learns about the patient from the patient. Respectful assessment of patient needs, beliefs about health care, and preferences for how that care is provided is essential. In most health-care settings, allowance for individual practices is possible when the practices are compatible with treatment guidelines. When that is not possible, education and discussion of options can result in acceptable solutions.

CLINICS CARE POINTS

- Approach all patients with respect using soft tones and when accepted, a handshake.
- Discreetly approach assessment of practices and needs. Indirect approaches to obtaining information are usually more acceptable.
- Listen carefully. Respect periods of silence because they may reflect consideration of what is being said.
- Direct eye contact may be avoided, sometimes in respect of an authority figure. Nonverbal behavior may indicate discomfort.
- Ceremonies, rituals, and the placement of objects near the patient may be important to a feeling of well-being and are often compatible with traditional medicine. When possible, allow these practices.
- Dietary restrictions and additions are common, and these aspects of care should be carefully assessed. Most hospitals have sources for foods specific to various cultures and religions. If not, the caregiver should discuss options with the patient and/or family.
- Patients may want to fast according to their religious practices; however, most religions provide options for when a person is ill.
- Just as traditional medications are reconciled on admission and discharge, the use of complementary or alternative substances should also be assessed and reconciled. Many institutions have integrated nontraditional approaches into routine care. However, there are substances and practices that may interfere with the prescribed treatments.
- Regardless of culture or religion, patients may prefer caregivers of the same gender.
- Respect for patient modesty is basic to the care of any patient. However, some patients may wish to wear specific garments including head coverings.
- When preparing patients for surgery or other procedures, the patients should understand that body hair, including head hair or beards may be removed. Head hair and beards may have significant importance to the patient.
- Patients may want any body organs or parts such as ribs to be cared for in a manner designated by their culture or religion. Some cultures bury the placenta after birth and some bury any removed body parts with the deceased person.

- Rituals and ceremonies surrounding birth and death are common and patients and families should be consulted before any decisions.
- The time and method of circumcision is specified for some religious groups and is often scheduled after the infant is discharged home.
- Care of the dying patient and care of the body after death vary by culture and religion. Patient and family preferences should be assessed before making any decisions.
- Inclusion of religious leaders, tribal elders, and possibly medicine men is often important to the patient and family. The presence of these figures is often calming for the patient and well incorporated into the routine care.

DISCLOSURE

The authors have nothing to disclose.

REFERENCES

1. Frisch NC, Rabinowitsch D. What's in a Definition? Holistic Nursing, Integrative Health Care, and Integrative Nursing: Report of an Integrated Literature Review. J Holist Nurs 2019;37(3):260–72.
2. Kagawa-Singer M. Impact of culture on health outcomes. J Pediatr Hematol On-col 2011;33(Suppl 2):S90–5.
3. M.G. White. 5 Main World Religions and Their Basic Beliefs. Your Dictionary. 2021 Available at: https://www.yourdictionary.com/articles/world-religions-beliefs. Accessed August 1, 2023.
4. Alch CK, Wright CL, Collier KM, et al. Barriers to Addressing the Spiritual and Religious Needs of Patients and Families in the Intensive Care Unit: A Qualitative Study of Critical Care Physicians. Am J Hosp Palliat Care 2021;38(9):1120–5.
5. Choi PJ, Curlin FA, Cox CE. Addressing religion and spirituality in the intensive care unit: A survey of clinicians. Palliat Support Care 2019;17(2):159–64.
6. Best MC, Vivat B, Gijsberts M-J. Spiritual Care in Palliative Care. Religions 2023; 14(3):320. https://doi.org/10.3390/rel14030320.
7. Alive. Culture and Death: Native American Heritage. Alive. 2021 https://www.alivehospice.org/news-events/culture-and-death-native-american-heritage/. Accessed August 1, 2023.
8. Clayton, D, Evans, AC. Native American Religions. Study.com. 2022. https://study.com/learn/lesson/native-american-religions-traditions-overview-history-beliefs.html. Accessed August 1, 2023.
9. Indian Health Service. Cultural Highlights for HIS Indian Health Professionals: A Reference Guide to American Indian and Alaska Native Culture. 2017. https://www.ihs.gov/sites/careeropps/themes/responsive2017/display_objects/documents/Cultural_ZCard.pdf. Accessed August 1, 2023.
10. Metropolitan Chicago Health Care Council (MCHC). Guidelines For Health Care Providers Interacting with American Indian (Native American; First Nation) Patients and Their Families. Advocate Health.com 2004;1–9. Accessed August 2, 2023.
11. Luna JAA, Moore R, Calac DJ, et al. Practices Surrounding Pain Management Among American Indians and Alaska Natives in Rural Southern California: An Exploratory Study. J Rural Health 2019;35(1):133–8.
12. Centgene Corporation. Culture and Heritage are Key to Tribal Community Health: Transforming Communities, Health & Wellness. Centgene.com. 2021, 2023.

https://www.centene.com/news/culture-and-heritage-key-to-tribal-community-health.html. Accessed August 3, 2023.

13. Koithan M, Farrell C. Indigenous Native American Healing Traditions. J Nurse Pract 2010;6(6):477–8. https://doi.org/10.1016/j.nurpra.2010.03.016.

14. Harley, M. Welcoming All Families: Supporting the Native American Family. Lamaze International. 2014. https://www.lamaze.org/Connecting-the-Dots/Post/series-welcoming-all-families-supporting-the-native-american-family. Accessed August 3, 2023.

15. Hayward A, Cidro J. Indigenous Birth as Ceremony and a Human Right. Health Hum Rights 2021;23(1):213–24.

16. Muza, S. Supporting the Native American Family: Connecting the Past and the Present. Lamaze International. 2014. https://www.lamaze.org/Connecting-the-Dots/Post/series-welcoming-all-families-supporting-the-native-american-family. Accessed August 3, 2023.

17. Anderson K. Life stages and native women. Winnipeg: University of Manitoba Press; 2011.

18. Pew Research Center. The size of the U.S. Jewish population. Pew Research.org. 2021 https://www.pewresearch.org/religion/2021/05/11/the-size-of-the-u-s-jewish-population/. Accessed August 5, 2023..

19. Alper, B.A., Cooperman, A. 10 key findings about Jewish Americans. Pew Research.org. 2021. Sccessed August 5, 2023. https://www.pewresearch.org/short-reads/2021/05/11/10-key-findings-about-jewish-americans/.

20. My Jewish Learning. The Jewish Denominations: A quick look at Reform, Conservative, Orthodox and Reconstructionist Judaism — and at Other Jewish Streams. My Jewish Learning. No date. https://www.myjewishlearning.com/article/the-jewish-denominations/. Accessed August 6, 2023.

21. Weiner J. Jewish Values in Medical Decision-making for Unrepresented Patients: A Ritualized Approach. Rambam Maimonides Med J 2021;12(3):e0023.

22. Lapsley, J. Spirituality in Medicine-Judaism. Indiana University School of Medicine: Spirit of Medicine. 2021. https://medicine.iu.edu/blogs/spirit-of-medicine/spirituality-in-medicine—judaism. Accessed August 5. 2023.

23. Jewish Visiting. Caring For A Jewish Patient - A Guide For Medical Professionals. Jewish Visiting. No Date. https://www.jvisit.org.uk/caring-for-a-jewish-patient-a-guide-for-medical-professionals/. Accessed August 4, 2023.

24. Rich, TR. Birth and the First Month of Life. Jewfaq.org. No Date https://www.jewfaq.org/birth. Accessed august 6, 2023.

25. Jewish virtual Library. (n.d.). Death & Bereavement in Judaism: Death and Mourning. Jewish virtual Library. No Date https://www.jewishvirtuallibrary.org/death-and-mourning-in-judaism. Accessed August 6, 2023.

26. Gallimore, D. Understanding Filipino Traits, values, and Culture. Outsourceaccelerator.com. 2023 https://www.outsourceaccelerator.com/articles/filipino-traits-and-values/. Accessed August 4, 2023.

27. Queensland Health. Filipino Australians. Queensland Health.qld.gov.au. 2011 https://www.health.qld.gov.au/__data/assets/pdf_file/0024/157650/filipino2011.pdf. Accessed August 7, 2023.

28. Stanford Medicine. Filipino American Older Adults. Geriatrics.Stanford.edu. 2010;1–15. Accessed August 3, 2023.

29. Queensland Health. Filipino Ethnicity and Background. Hlth,qld.Gov.Au. No ate. Accessed August 1, 2023.

30. Jimenez, MT. Death and Dying: A Filipino American Perspective. Diverse Elders. 2019. https://diverseelders.org/2019/12/03/death-and-dying-a-filipino-american-perspective/. Accessed August 3, 2023.
31. Times Prayer. The number of Muslims around the World. Times Prayer. 2023. https://timesprayer.com/en/muslim-population/. Accessed August 3, 2023.
32. Council on American Islamic Relations. A health Care Providers to Islamic Religious Practices. Council on American Islamic Relations. 2005. https://www.cair.com/wp-content/uploads/2020/02/A-Health-Care-Provider%E2%80%99s-Guide-to-Islamic-Religious-Practices.pdf. Accessed August 4. 2023.
33. Mataoui FZ, Sheldon LK. Providing Culturally Appropriate Care to American Muslims With Cancer. Clin J Oncol Nurs 2016;20(1):11–3. https://doi.org/10.1188/16. CJON.11-12.
34. Queensland Government/Queensland Health. Health Care Providers' Handbook on Muslim Patients. Queensland Health. 2013. https://www.health.qld.gov.au/multicultural/health_workers/hbook-muslim. Accessed August 7, 2023.
35. Gatrad, AR, Sheikh, A. Muslim Birth Customs. Archives of Disease in Childhood - Fetal and Neonatal Edition; 2001;84:F6-F8. https://fn.bmj.com/content/84/1/F6.info.
36. United States Census Bureau. Quick Facts: Hispanic or Latino. United States Census Bureau. 2023. https://www.census.gov/quickfacts/fact/table/US/RHI725222. Accessed August 1, 2023.
37. Fowler AL, Mann ME, Martinez FJ, et al. Cultural Health Beliefs and Practices Among Hispanic Parents. Clin Pediatr 2022;61(1):56–65. https://doi.org/10.1177/00099228211059666.
38. Moslimani, M, Lopez, MH, Noe-Bustamante, L. 11 facts about Hispanic origin groups in the U.S. Pew Research Center. 2023. https://www.pewresearch.org/short-reads/2023/08/16/11-facts-about-hispanic-origin-groups-in-the-us/. Accessed October 16, 2023.
39. Gast J, Peak T, Hunt A. Latino Health Behavior: An Exploratory Analysis of Health Risk and Health Protective Factors in a Community Sample. Am J Lifestyle Med 2017;14(1):97–106.
40. Nuñez A, González P, Talavera GA, et al. Machismo, Marianismo, and Negative Cognitive-Emotional Factors: Findings From the Hispanic Community Health Study/Study of Latinos Sociocultural Ancillary Study. J Lat Psychol 2016 Nov; 4(4):202–17.
41. Maternidad Latina. On Fertile Ground: Latina Health Beliefs During Pregnancy. Healthy Start Foundation. 2007. http://www.nchealthystart.org/aboutus/maternidad/vol1no2.htm. Accessed August 3, 2023.
42. Montoya-Williams D, Williamson VG, Cardel M, et al. The Hispanic/Latinx Perinatal Paradox in the United States: A Scoping Review and Recommendations to Guide Future Research. J Immigr Minority Health 2021;23(5):1078–91. https://doi.org/10.1007/s10903-020-01117-z.
43. Nomad Naturopath. Rue and Lavender Infused Hot Chocolate. Nomad Naturopath. 2020. https://nomadnaturopath.wordpress.com/2020/01/22/rue-and-lavender-infused-hot-chocolate/. Accessed August 3, 2023.
44. Gonzalez-Swafford MJ, Gutierrez MG. Ethno-medical beliefs and practices of Mexican Americans. Nurs Pract 1983;8(10):29–30, 32, 34.
45. Hohl S, Thompson B, Escareño M, et al. Cultural Norms in Conflict: Breastfeeding Among Hispanic Immigrants in Rural Washington State. Matern Child Health J 2016;20(7):1549–57.
46. Lopez, T. 10 Curious Customs of Latina Moms. Mom Life. 2013. https://mom.com/momlife/6602-10-curious-customs-latina-moms. Accessed August 6, 2023.

47. Cann, CK. Grief and Cultural Competence: Hispanic Traditions. No Date. https://funeralcourse.com/wp-content/uploads/2016/02/FSA-G-and-CC-H-1-WEB.pdf. Accessed august 7, 2023.
48. Office of Minority Health. Organ Donation and Hispanic Americans. Health and Human Services. 2021. https://minorityhealth.hhs.gov/omh/browse.aspx?lvl=4&lvlid=72. Accessed august 7, 2023.

Interprofessional Education and Essential Approach to Health care

Blanca Iris Padilla, PhD, MBA, APRN, MSN, FNP-BC, FAANP

KEYWORDS

- Interprofessional education • Interprofessional collaborative care • Team-based care
- Nursing leaders

KEY POINTS

- Nursing leaders?
- Interprofessional education is the key to improving patient safety.
- Interprofessional collaboration is crucial for best practice and patient outcomes.
- Interprofessional education and collaboration is patient-centered.

INTRODUCTION

The US health care system has a history of being costly, fragmented, unreliable, and reactive, thus contributing to and sustaining health disparities.[1] Interprofessional education and collaboration (IPEC) have long been recognized and proliferated in academic and health care organizations as an approach that can provide transparency and quality effective health care with optimal outcomes to individuals, families, and communities. A national paradigm shift toward well-organized interprofessional collaborative teams is underway but requires diverse health care providers with shared goals and values to work together to provide safe, efficient, timely, patient-centered comprehensive care. This article provides a historical perspective on IPEC and discusses this approach to patient care.

HISTORY AND DEFINITIONS

In 1972, the Institute of Medicine (IOM; now the National Academy of Medicine [NAM]) released a landmark report entitled "Educating for the Health Team,"[2] which introduced the concept of using a team to deliver efficient, effective, competent patient care. It was suggested that a team approach would optimize the knowledge and skills

Duke University School of Nursing, Duke University Health System, DUMC 3322, 307 Trent Drive, Durham, NC 27707, USA
E-mail address: iris.padilla@duke.edu

Nurs Clin N Am 59 (2024) 37–47
https://doi.org/10.1016/j.cnur.2023.11.005
0029-6465/24/© 2023 Elsevier Inc. All rights reserved.
nursing.theclinics.com

of members and, importantly, include patients in the team, thus allowing them to participate in decision-making pertaining to their well-being.[2] Nonetheless, by the turn of the century, IOM committee reports[3,4] were documenting extensive concerns regarding quality, safety, and errors in the US health care system. One report in particular, *To Err is Human: Building a Safer Health System*,[3] was instrumental in raising awareness of issues including, but not limited to, substandard services, long waiting times, delays, and waste, thus setting the tone and impetus to improve patient care in the UShealth care system.

In 2001, an IOM report recommended that an interprofessional summit be held to develop strategies to restructure clinical education for all health professionals with the specific aim of enhancing care quality and meeting the needs of the country's diverse population. The Committee on the Health Professions Education Summit was held in 2002 and attended by 150 participants from diverse health professions, including educators, students, and other representatives from allied health, nursing, medicine, pharmacology, and health professional industries. The committee's ensuing report, *Health Professions Education: A Bridge to* Quality,[5] recommended 5 core competencies (ie, patient-centered care, interdisciplinary teams, evidence-based practice, quality improvement, informatics) for health professions education, and oversight and credentialing processes to ensure that interdisciplinary teams could function efficiently and effectively.

Defining Interprofessional Education

In 1997, the Center for the Advancement of Interprofessional Education (CAIPE) established a globally accepted definition for interprofessional education (IPE), which was modified in 2002 as follows: "Occasions when two or more professions learn with, from and about each other to improve collaboration and the quality of care."[6] CAIPE modified this definition again in 2016, adding, "to improve collaboration and quality of care and services."[7] The World Health Organization (WHO) offers a similar definition for IPE, and the most widely used: "When students from two or more professions learn about, from, and with each other to enable effective collaboration and improve health outcomes."[8] These definitions of IPE reflect concepts and practices of interprofessional health and social care which propelled interactions among members of different professions beyond merely working in a shared environment[8] and thus were precursors for Interprofessional Collaborative Practice (IPCP).[9] Interprofessional education is now considered an essential component of health professions education because it (a) supports the delivery of effective care, and (b) addresses the current complexities of health care systems and health system policies.

BACKGROUND
Interprofessional Collaborative Practice: Emergence Toward Competency Domains

By 2009, despite a decade of committee reports and recommendations regarding IPE and interdisciplinary team competencies, representatives of 6 national associations of schools of the health professions concurred that IPE was not translating into interprofessional collaborative practices that could sufficiently address health system quality and safety issues.[10] In 2010, they convened an expert panel of educators from various health professions to develop discipline-specific core competencies for interprofessional collaborative practices grounded on the IOM core competencies to promote better patient care and more person-centered, community-centered, and population-centered health care systems. In 2011, the IPEC expert panel (**Box 1**) established 4 competency domains with specific sub-competency objectives and

---

Box 1
IPEC Expert Panel

2011 Expert Panel
  American Association of Colleges of Nursing
  American Association of Colleges of Osteopathic Medicine
  American Association of Colleges of Pharmacy
  American Dental Education Association
  Association of American Medical Colleges
  Association of Schools of Public Health

2016 Additional Experts
  American Association of Colleges of Podiatric Medicine
  American Council of Academic Physical Therapy,
  American Occupational Therapy Association,
  American Psychological Association,
  Association of American Veterinary Medical Colleges
  Association of Schools and Colleges of Optometry
  Association of Schools of Allied Health Professions,
  Council on Social Work Education
  Physician Assistant Education Association

---

assessments of (1) values/ethics for interprofessional practice, (2) roles/responsibilities, (3) interprofessional communication, and (4) teams and teamwork[10]; these were updated in 2016 to reflect changes in health systems and the implementation of the Patient Protection and Affordable Care Act.[6]

The current draft of *The IPEC Core Competencies: 2023 Update*[7] retains the same domains, significantly revises sub-competencies (including some deletions and additions), and incorporates language that emphasizes inclusivity, cultural humility, team science, and health outcomes (**Table 1** for details). Importantly, the newly proposed subcompetency statements integrate terms such as "culture, cultural humility, and social determinants of health (SDOH) and health outcomes."[7] Culture is a construct that impacts health and health-seeking behavior; therefore, the inclusion of these terms represents a major paradigm shift toward improving population health and health inequities. The complexity of SDOH is well documented in the literature and best addressed by an interprofessional workforce that includes non-medical professionals (eg, social workers, insurance navigators, attorneys)[11] able to navigate and address obstacles. The current competencies reflect an awareness that teams must function and communicate efficiently, and their members must share goals, mutual trust, and an understanding of one another's roles in order to effect needed changes.

The 2015 National Academy of Medicine's (NAM) report on IPE and IPEC emphasized the need to demonstrate an association between IPE and collaborative practice and patient outcomes, and provided guidelines for designing, analyzing, and reporting studies on IPE across the health professions learning continuum.[12] A 2016 summary of the report[13] highlighted the following key elements.

- Findings of the literature reviewed show that IPE can improve learner's knowledge, skills, and understanding of IPE practice, but limited empirical data linking IPE practice to patient, population, and health system outcomes
- Lack of taxonomy or conceptual model tying educational interventions to learning, patient health, or health system outcomes
- Inconsistency in the IPE environment and extensive lag time between some interventions and outcomes.

Table 1 The IPEC core competencies: 2023 update	
Emerging 2023 Core Competencies and Definitions	2023 Emerging Subcompetencies
Values and Ethics: Work with team members to maintain a climate of shared values, ethical conduct, and mutual respect.	Promote the values and interests of persons and populations in health care delivery, One Health, and population health initiatives. [a]Advocate for social justice and health equity of persons and populations across the lifespan. Uphold the dignity, privacy, identity, and autonomy of persons while maintaining confidentiality in the delivery of team-based care. Value diversity, identities, cultures, and differences. Value the expertise of health professionals and its impact on team functions and health outcomes. Collaborate with honesty and integrity while striving for health equity and improvements in health outcomes. Practice trust, empathy, respect, and compassion with persons, caregivers, health professionals, and populations. Apply high standards of ethical conduct and quality in contributions to team-based care. Maintain competence in one's own profession in order to contribute to interprofessional care. [a]Contribute to a just culture that fosters self-fulfillment, collegiality, and civility across the team. [a]Support a workplace where differences are respected, career satisfaction is supported, and well-being is prioritized.
Roles and Responsibilities: *Use the knowledge of one's own role and team members' expertise to address health outcomes.*	Practice cultural humility in interprofessional teamwork. Incorporate complementary expertise to meet health needs including the social determinants of health. Include the full scope of knowledge, skills, and attitudes of team members to provide care that is person-centered, safe, cost-effective, timely, efficient, effective, and equitable. Differentiate each team member's role, scope of practice, and responsibility in promoting health outcomes. Collaborate with others within and outside of the health system to improve health outcomes.

(continued on next page)

Table 1 (continued)	
Emerging 2023 Core Competencies and Definitions	**2023 Emerging Subcompetencies**
Communication: Communicate in a responsive, responsible, respectful, and compassionate manner with team members.	Use communication tools, techniques, and technologies to enhance team function, well-being, and health outcomes. Communicate clearly with authenticity and cultural humility, avoiding discipline-specific terminology. Promote common understanding and teamwork toward shared goals. Practice active listening that encourages ideas and opinions of other team members. Use constructive feedback to connect, align, and accomplish team goals. Examine one's position, power, hierarchical role, unique experience, expertise, and culture toward improving communication and managing conflicts. [a]Communicate one's roles and responsibilities clearly.
Teams and Teamwork: Apply values and principles of team science to adapt one's own role in a variety of team settings.	Describe evidence-informed processes of team development and practices. Apply interprofessional conflict management methods, including identifying conflict cause and addressing divergent perspectives. Share team accountability for outcomes. Reflect on self and team performance to inform and improve team effectiveness. [a]Facilitate care coordination to achieve safe, effective care, and health outcomes. [a]Operate from a shared framework that supports resiliency, well-being, safety, and efficacy. [a]Discuss organizational structures, policies, practices, resources, access to information, and timing issues that impact the effectiveness of the team. [a]Appreciate team members' diverse experiences, expertise, cultures, positions, power, and hierarchical roles toward improving team function.

[a] Denotes newly added.
Adapted from Interprofessional Education Collaborative. (2023). IPEC Core Competencies for Interprofessional Collaborative Practice: Version 3. Washington, DC: Interprofessional Education Collaborative.

The report committee's recommendations included resources for well-designed studies and optimization of study designs, including mixed methods (quantitative and qualitative); however, missing from this report were references to culture competence, population health and literacy inequities, and SDOH.

In addition to the NAM's 2015 report, the National Center Data Repository provides health care organizations and academic institutions with evidence-based resources on how IPE and IPEC may improve health care and population health, and decrease health care cost.[14] However, despite national recommendations, IPE research designs continue to lack consistency, quality, and vigor.[15] Moreover, designs are lacking that measure the interrelationships between SDOH and health outcomes, an important factor to understanding health equity.[16]

Interprofessional Education and Collaborative Practice

The Framework for Action on Interprofessional Education and Collaborative Practice[9] was created by the WHOStudy Group on IPE and IPEC in response to an urgent global shortage of health care workers (**Fig. 1**). Two of its key messages were that "interprofessional collaboration in education and practice [is] an innovative strategy that will play an important role in mitigating the global health workforce crisis," and "interprofessional education is a necessary step in preparing a 'collaborative practice-ready health workforce."[9(p7)] Several of its stated recognitions are worth noting: (1) many health systems globally are fragmented, (2) health-services providers face increasingly complex health issues, and (3) a collaborative practice-ready workforce can mitigate health system fragmentation and improve health services and health outcomes.[9(p10)] Despite the framework's assertion that "if health workforce planning and policymaking are integrated, interprofessional education and collaborative practice can be fully supported,"[9(p10)] the fostering of IPE and clinical practice experiences has remained limited in academia.[17]

Interprofessional learning experiences prepare health professions students to provide team-based care[18] but may be hindered by limited physical space, course availability/timing, and other logistical challenges, or resistance to change. For example, Thistlethwaite (2015) has described numerous considerations involved when introducing IPE into medical school curricula.[19] The development of IPE clinical experiences for health professions students should be well-planned and intentional, with buy-in from all key stakeholders, including, but not limited to, health care organization administrators and academic leaders.

One example of effective IPEC is a direct observation clinical experience with feedback in real-time that was created in an emergency department (ED) at a large academic health system for health professions students from the schools of medicine, nursing, and physical therapy.[20] Clinical sessions were led by trained interprofessional faculty in an IPE clinic space near the ED that was not occupied at night. Interprofessional faculty facilitated clinical sessions and engaged in teaching while providing direct observation to health professions students (medicine, nursing, physical therapy, and physician assistant) engaged in team-based patient care in the IPE clinic. Prior to

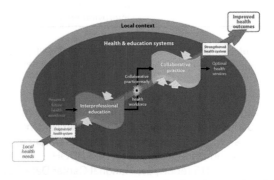

Fig. 1. Framework for Action on Interprofessional Education and Collaborative Practice World Health Organization, 2010.

the start of the clinical sessions, team members introduced themselves and developed a plan of care plan, which was communicated to the patient by the IPE faculty and team. In addition to addressing patients' reasons for visiting the ED, students assessed for emotional, cultural-socioeconomic, and environmental barriers to care, and referred patients to appropriate community resources as part of their management plan. At the end of the clinical session, students were provided real-time feedback and an evaluation.

An important aspect of this experience was a faculty-student dialogue regarding reasons that patients had elected to seek care in the ED (eg, uninsured status, no primary care provider, perceived illness).[20] Discussions on social needs and lack of community resources in disadvantaged groups provided health professions students with insights into health-seeking behaviors, SDOH, and health inequities. Feedback data showed that most students considered the IPE experience positive and the environment respectful. Patients who elected to be seen at the IPE clinic reported higher satisfaction than those who remained at the ED.[20] Similarly, the IPE faculty and leadership team displayed consistency and dedication, shared their appreciation for the opportunity to teach and learn from one another, and attended faculty development sessions. Overall, this experience illustrates a collaborative team-based approach to health care education and practice.

Today's health professions students will likely practice well into the twenty-first century and will need to meet changing health service demands and needs[19] as well as demonstrate flexibility in thinking and responding while working in teams. Team-based learning in an IPE environment promotes this flexibility through mutual learning and the development of plans that address health care problems in their complexity.[21]

DISCUSSION

It is well documented in the literature that there is no one health profession that can meet patients' needs; future health professionals must be prepared to learn not only "with" but "from" and "about" one another.[19] In fact, given the increase in health care complexity and patients with multiple chronic conditions, it is not only challenging to be the sole provider of care but also potentially unsafe.[22] IPEC has become integral and necessary to health professions education, practice, and health care. Health care delivery must be patient-centered and should be delivered by a multidisciplinary team who understand one another's roles and responsibilities and communicate and collaborate effectively. For example, a recent IPE study exploring health profession students' experience in interprofessional practice managing patients with type 2 diabetes showed that health professions students reported the value of their IPE learning experience and delivery of patient-centered care as a team versus the traditional single-provider approach that often drives the patient-provider interview.[23] This is one of many examples of the growing need for and appreciation of collaboration among health care professionals for best practice and patient outcomes.

As IPE and IPEC incorporate new sub-competencies about inclusivity, cultural humility, social justice, and SDOH with a strong focus on team science and collaboration, it is important to emphasize that nurses are well-positioned to lead work within interprofessional teams in health care organizations. It is also worth noting that, historically, nurses have been and continue to be at the forefront of patient care and a strong presence in various settings and roles within and beyond the health care industry. Additionally, nurses have proven to be change agents who are instrumental in developing structures and policies that bridge health care systems and social needs for individuals, families, and communities.

SUMMARY

The changing landscape of today's US health care system calls for a different approach in care delivery. To adequately address the health care challenges, and improve patients' outcomes, while reducing the per capita cost of health care, key stakeholders such as academic and health care leaders must come together to provide health profession students interprofessional learning opportunities that include didactic and authentic clinical training to become a practice-ready member of today's health care workforce. Additionally, faculty and health professionals teaching IPE must engage in ongoing faculty development and serve as role models. Finally, the significance of the inclusion of SDOH, culture, cultural humility, and social justice in the IPEC 2023 core competencies cannot be overemphasized. All health care professionals must work together and develop strategies that break down the silos and barriers and address health inequities.

CLINICS CARE POINTS

The emergence of IPE and IPEC has led to a paradigm shift in health professions education and health care delivery. Team-based learning in an IPE environment allows students to develop flexibility in thinking while working with team members to find solutions to complex health care problems.[21] Below are listed some of the relevant clinical practice points based on the literature and the author's expertise. Although these evidence-based practice pearls and pitfalls are noted in the literature, their integration and operationalization may vary depending on the organization, academic setting, and health care system.

Pearls
- Establish and/or enhance academic-practice partnerships with mutual goals that
  ○ Provide a setting in which health professions students can meet IPEC core competencies and sub-competencies
  ○ Offer an environment in which learning is intentional and authentic[23,24]
  ○ Allow health professions students opportunities to work together and contribute to teams[25]
- Provide faculty with professional development: Faculty involved or interested in IPE and IPEC should engage in ongoing professional development. Relevant topics may include
  ○ IPEC Core Competencies[7]
  ○ Understanding characteristics and structure of team[7]
  ○ Communication and collaboration[26]
  ○ Providing and receiving feedback[26]
  ○ Team precepting and mentoring[15,26,27]
- All patient care must be patient-centered. This is one of the subcompetencies of IPEC. The IPE team must inform the patient and discuss with them that team-based care is a new model of care.[20,26]
- Health professionals working in effective interprofessional teams can provide safe, quality patient-centered care and navigate complex health care settings.[28]
- Integrate SDOH into clinical experiential learning. Optimal health outcomes cannot be achieved without addressing barriers to care. Addressing SDOH is in alignment with the IPEC Core Competencies.[10,15]

Pitfalls
- Pitfalls or challenges to implementing IPE and IPEC are well documented in the literature. Some of the most common are
  ○ the traditional culture of physician dominance in the health care industry[15,29]
  ○ intraprofessional conflict[29]
  ○ logistics and time constraints among students and providers[30]

- lack of faculty development[31]
- lack of or inadequate resources[20]
- lack of communication skills and strategies[30,32]

DISCLOSURE

The author does not have anything to disclose.

REFERENCES

1. Earnest M, Brandt B. Aligning practice redesign and interprofessional education to advance triple aim outcomes. J Interprof Care 2014;28(6):497–500.
2. National Center for Interprofessional Practice and Education. Institute of Medicine. Educating for the health team. Washington, DC: National Academy of Sciences; 1972. Available at: https://nexusipe.org/informing/resource-center/iom-1972-report-educating-health-team.
3. Institute of Medicine (US). In: Kon LT, Corrgan JM, Donaldson MS, editors. Committee on quality of healthcare in America. To Err is human: building a safer health system. Washington (DC): National Academies Press (US); 2000. Available at: https://www.ncbi.nlm.nih.gov/books/NBK225182/PMID. Accessed on July 10, 2023.
4. Institute of Medicine (US). Committee on quality of healthcare in America. Crossing the quality chasm: a new health system for the 21st century. Washington (DC): National Academies Press (US); 2001. Available at: https://www.ncbi.nlm.nih.gov/books/NBK222274/.
5. Institute of Medicine (US). Committee on the Health Professions Education Summit. In: Greiner AC, Knebel E, editors. Health professions education: a bridge to quality. Washington (DC): National Academies Press (US); 2003. Available at: https://www.ncbi.nlm.nih.gov/books/NBK221528/.
6. Barr H. CAIPE-2002-Interprofessional Education: Today, Yesterday, and Tomorrow. Center for Advancement of Interprofessional Education (CAIPE). Available at: https://www.caipe.org/resources/publications/caipe-publications/caipe-2002-interprofessional-education-today-yesterday-tomorrow-barr-hhttp://www.caipe.org.uk.
7. Interprofessional Education Collaborative. Preamble, definition, assumptions, and tenets of IPEC's 2021-2023 core competency revision (CCR) working group. 2022 interprofessional collaborative practice. Washington, DC: Interprofessional Education Collaborative; 2023.
8. World Health Organization. Framework for Action on Interprofessional Education & Collaboration Practice. 2010. Reference number: WHO/HRH/HPN/10.3. Available at: https://www.who.int/publications/i/item/framework-for-action-on-interprofessional-education-collaborative-practice
9. Headrick LA, Wilcock PM, Batalden PB. Interprofessional working and continuing medical education. BMJ 1998;316:771–4.
10. Schmitt M, Blue A, Aschenbrener CA, et al. Core competencies for interprofessional collaborative practice: reforming healthcare by transforming health professionals' education. Acad Med 2011;86:1351.
11. Association of Academic Health Centers. Academic health centers and social determinants of health: challenges & barriers, responses & solutions. AAHC Social Determinants of Health Initiative; 2015. Available at: https://www.aamc.org/. Accessed August 3, 2023.

12. National Academy of Medicine. Measuring the impact on interprofessional and collaborative practice and patient outcomes. Washington D.C: . The National Academies Press; 2015. Available at: https://nap.nationalacademies.org/catalog/21726/measuring-the-impact-of-interprofessional-education-on-collaborative-practice-and-patient-outcomes.

13. Cox M, Cuff P, Brandt B, et al. Measuring the impact of interprofessional education on collaborative practice and outcomes. J Interprof Care 2016;30(1):1–3.

14. Pechacek J, Shanedling J, Lutfiyya MN, et al. The national United States Center data repository: Core essential interprofessional practice & education data enabling triple aim analytics. J Interprof Care 2015;29(6):587–91.

15. Thibault GE. The future of health professional education: Emerging trends in the U.S. FASEB BioAdvances 2020;2:685–94.

16. Dover DC, Belon AP. The health equity measurement framework; a comprehensive model to measure social inequities in health. Int J Equity Health 2019;18(36):1–2.

17. Mohammed CA, Anand R, Ummer VS. Interprofessional education (IPE): a framework for introducing teamwork and collaboration in health professions curriculum. Med J Armed Forces India 2021;77(S1):S16–21.

18. Zorek JA, Lacy J, Gaspard C, et al. Leveraging the interprofessional education collaborative competency framework to transform health professions education. Am J Pharmaceut Educ 2021;85(7):8602.

19. Thistlethwaite JE. Interprofessional education: implications and development for medical education. Educ Méd 2015;16(1):68–73. Available at: http://creativecommons.org/licenses/by-nc-nd/4.0/.

20. Clay AS, Leiman ER, Theiling BJ, et al. Creating a win-win for the health system and health profession's education: a direct observation clinical experience with feedback iN real-time (DOCENT) for low acuity patients in the emergency room. BMC Med Educ 2022;66(1):1–11.

21. Meleis AI. Interprofessional education: a summary of reports and barriers to recommendations. J Nurs Scholarsh 2016;48(1):106–12.

22. Mitchell P, Wynia M, Golden R, et al. Core principles and values of effective team-based care. Washington, DC: National Academy of Medicine; 2012 [October, 12, 2012]. (Discussion Paper). Available at: https://nam.edu/perspectives-2012-core-principles-values-of-effective-team-based-health-care/.

23. Naumann F, Mullin R, Cawte A, et al. Designing, implementing and sustaining IPE within an authentic clinical environment: the impact on student learning. J Interprof Care 2021;35(6):907–13.

24. Lie D, Forest C, Kysh L, et al. 2016 Interprofessional education and practice guide No. 5: interprofessional teaching for prequalification students in clinical setting. J Interprof Care 2016;30(3):324–30.

25. Hickey M, Stillo M, Marquez C. An interprofessional clinical experience to address social determinants of health. J Am Acad Nurse Pract 2023;00:1–9.

26. Shrader S, Zaudke J. Top ten best practices for interprofessional precepting. Journal of Interprofessional Education & Practice 2018;10:56–60.

27. Kreider KE, Rowell JV, Bowers M, et al. Effective interprofessional precepting in a specialty clinic: utilizing evidence and lived experiences to optimize the trainer of diverse learners. Journal of Interprofessional Education & Practice 2022;26:100490.

28. Kowalski K. Creating interprofessional teams. J Cont Educ Nurs 2018;49(7):297–8.

29. Apold S, Pohl JM. No turning back. J Nurse Pract 2014;10(2):94–9.

30. Bollen A, Harrison R, Aslani P, et al. Factors influencing interprofessional collaboration between community pharmacists and general practitioners-A systematic review. Health Soc Care Community 2019;27(4):e189–212.
31. Dow A, Thibault G. Interprofessional education – A foundation for a new approach to healthcare. N Engl J Med 2017;377(9):803–4.
32. Rosen MA, DiazGranados D, Dieta AS, et al. Teamwork in healthcare: Key discoveries enabling safer, high-quality care. Am Psychol 2018;73(4):433–50.

Stress First Aid for Healthcare Workers

An Indicated Mental Illness Prevention Program for Nursing Education

Sean P. Convoy, DNP, PMHNP-BC[a],*, Mitchell Heflin, MD, MHS[b,c,d],
Bernice M. Alston, PhD[d], Undi Hoffler, PhD[e], Mary Barzee, MEd[d],
Julie Anne Thompson, PhD[d],
Richard Westphal, PhD, RN, PMHCNS-BC, PMHNP-BC[f]

KEYWORDS

- Stress First Aid for Healthcare Workers • Indicated mental illness prevention
- Peer support • Stress continuum • 4 sources of orange zone stress • Stress injury

KEY POINTS

- Stress First Aid for Healthcare Workers is a Basic Life Support for Stress initiative that relies on peer support to elevate community awareness around stress-related injury and illness designed to preserve life, prevent further harm, and promote recovery.
- The Stress Continuum serves as an organizing framework from which community members can measure and classify how both self and others may be responding to stress.
- The 4 Sources of Orange Zone Stress (eg, trauma, loss, inner conflict, and wear and tear) are unique forms of stress that confer a greater risk for orange zone and red zone behaviors.
- The stress first aid model is an alliterative preclinical framework defined by the 7 C's (eg, check, coordinate, cover, calm, connect, competence, and confidence) designed to operationalize how one peer responds to another experiencing stress.

[a] School of Nursing, Duke University, 307 Trent Drive, Durham, NC 27710, USA; [b] Center for Interprofessional Education and Care (IPEC), Duke University, 307 Trent Drive, Durham, NC 27710, USA; [c] Division of Geriatrics, Duke University School of Medicine, Aging Center at Duke, Geriatric Evaluation and Treatment Clinic, 307 Trent Drive, Durham, NC 27710, USA; [d] Duke University School of Nursing, DUMC 33223, 307 Trent Drive, Durham, NC 27700, USA; [e] North Carolina Central University, 1801 Fayetteville Street, Durham, NC 27707, USA; [f] Family, Community & Mental Health Systems, University of Virginia School of Nursing, 225 Jeanette Lancaster Way, Charlottesville, VA 22903, USA
* Corresponding author. Duke University School of Nursing, DUMC 3322, 3307 Trent Drive, Durham, NC 27700.
E-mail address: sean.convoy@duke.edu

Nurs Clin N Am 59 (2024) 49–61
https://doi.org/10.1016/j.cnur.2023.11.006
0029-6465/24/© 2023 Elsevier Inc. All rights reserved.

nursing.theclinics.com

NATURE OF THE PROBLEM

According to a survey published by Mental Health America and funded by the Johnson & Johnson Foundation, 93% of health-care workers are experiencing clinically significant and functionally impairing symptoms of stress, anxiety, frustration intolerance, sadness, anger, fear, grief, impaired sleep, changes in appetite, and somatic symptoms.[1] Recent research suggests that up to 40% of health-care professionals will struggle with a trauma and stressor-related disorder following the coronavirus disease 2019 (COVID-19) pandemic.[2] A 2023 AMN Healthcare survey identified that 30% of the 18,000 Registered Nurse (RNs) surveyed indicated that they are likely to leave the profession due to the pandemic and its lingering sequelae.[3] Health professions students and trainees likewise are prone to higher rates of stress and burnout than age-matched peers in the general population.[4,5] This is associated with higher rates of depressive symptoms and seems to have worsened during the pandemic and concurrent social strife related to long-standing systemic biases.[6,7] Since COVID-19, 5.5% of American nurses have contemplated suicide and were regrettably reluctant to engage in care.[8] Considered individually, each statistical represents a concerning trend. Considered together, the data represent a genuine crisis.

Traditionally, occupational stressors in health care include common factors, such as long work hours, high clinical acuity and patient volume, intense physical and emotional labor, and exposure to human suffering. Recently, new and evolving psychosocial stressors such as COVID-19 sequelae, acute and/or chronic racial and social injustice, and political and economic instability have contributed to unprecedented exposure to *trauma*, *loss*, *inner conflict*, and *wear* and *tear*. COVID-19 has revealed critical deficiencies in traditional strategies to both recognize and respond to occupational stress within the health-care setting.

Because it relates to occupational stress within health care, a polarization of explanations and responsibility exists between health-care management and health-care workers. Health-care management commonly rebrands the impacts of occupational stress through the prism of personal resiliency. Alternatively, health-care workers are more inclined to view occupational stress through the lens of those complicating stressors unique to the work setting. The National Institute for Occupational Safety and Health[9] defines occupational stress as, *"the harmful physical and emotional responses that occur when the requirements of the job do not match the capabilities, resources, or needs of the worker."* Embracing the dialectic, both perspectives are true. Health-care workers do have a responsibility to champion their own mental health and health-care managers also shoulder the responsibility to actively surveil and remediate those modifiable risk factors in the workspace that breed unnecessary stress. As tensions with health-care systems increase, the incidence and prevalence of stress among the health-care workforce insensibly robs nurses of their capacity to serve and care. We are long overdue for a paradigm change where peer support is championed to counter stress in the health-care workspace.

CONCEPTUAL FRAMEWORKS
Mrazek and Haggerty's Model of the Spectrum of Interventions for Mental Health Problems and Mental Disorders

Figure 1 depicts Mrazek and Haggerty's Model of the Spectrum of Interventions for Mental Health Problems and Mental Disorders.[10] Envisioning the mental health-care system through the model, the line of clinical significance where formal systems of mental health care are commonly engaged is in the space between *indicated prevention* and *case identification*. From a health-care delivery system perspective, those

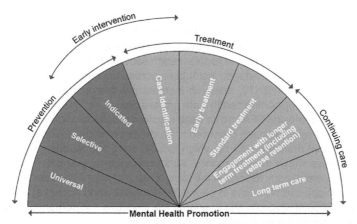

Fig. 1. Mrazek and Haggerty's model of the spectrum of interventions for mental health problems and mental disorders. (Institute of Medicine. 1994. Reducing Risks for Mental Disorders: Frontiers for Preventive Intervention Research. https://doi.org/10.17226/2139. Reproduced with permission from the National Academy of Sciences, Courtesy of the National Academies Press, Washington, D.C.)

symptoms and stressors that exist below *case identification* are commonly not considered clinically significant. Generations of health-care providers have been trained to pay attention and respond to clinically significant symptoms using assessment, screening, and evaluation measures, which creates a bias for acuity and chronicity and against subclinical symptom recognition.

Mitigating this bias requires a new language to describe occupational stress within health care. Navigating COVID-19 as a health-care worker has been unquestionably stressful. Not all who experience this stress will manifest symptoms of mental illness such as acute stress disorder (ASD) or posttraumatic stress disorder (PTSD). Lifetime prevalence estimates for PTSD are estimated at 6.8%.[11] Using World Mental Health Survey data, cross-national lifetime prevalence of PTSD was 3.9% in the total sample and 5.6% among the trauma-exposed.[12] This evidence suggests not all who are exposed to trauma are destined to manifest a trauma and stressor-related disorder. New language is needed that codifies stress-related symptoms that exist below the line of clinical significance. The term "stress injury" is used as a preclinical term to recognize individuals who are subclinically responding to both the acute and chronic impacts of stress.[13] The relationship between a trauma and stressor-related disorder and stress injury is as follows: *All who meet diagnostic criteria for a trauma and stressor-related disorder (eg, ASD and PTSD) have encountered a stress injury but not all who have encountered a stress injury will necessarily manifest a trauma and stressor-related disorder.* The use of this new language is not merely an academic exercise. The introduction of the subclinical term *stress injury* creates an opportunity for us to look below the historical line of clinical significance intent to avoid exceeding it and creating an opportunity for mental health promotion and mental illness prevention.

Stress First Aid for Healthcare Workers Doctrine

Stress first aid (SFA) is an indicated mental illness prevention measure published by the National Center for PTSD,[14] which is largely based on the seminal research of S. E. Hobfoll and colleagues.[15,16] The Department of Navy and Marine Corps translated SFA into its established mental illness prevention doctrine in the form of Combat and

Operational Stress First Aid dating back to 2010.[13] Similarly, the Department of Veteran Affairs has also implemented the SFA framework into its organizational framework for mental illness prevention. Since then, there has been steady progress attempting to translate SFA doctrine beyond the federal health sector into first responder units,[17,18] health systems,[19–21] and academic institutions across the country.[21–24]

In the shadow of COVID-19, research increasingly demonstrates that SFA has a value-added role in supporting health-care professionals.[21,23,24] Currently, the University of Virginia is deploying SFA into its health system in collaboration with its School of Nursing. This content has been delivered to students on matriculation and conceptualized as a shared mental model by which faculty, staff, and students talk about and respond to stress within the community. Although outcome evaluation has not been published at present, early reports in the form of student evaluations are encouraging. In our case, an opportunity exists to gauge the favorability and impact of SFA across a diverse population of students and to adapt case vignettes and content to match more closely the needs of the evolving health-care worker.

Because SFA was produced using federal funding and resides in the public domain, SFA may be copied and distributed without permission. In sum, the evidence suggests that SFA is an effective preclinical strategy to conduct a timely assessment and preclinical response to suspected psychological injuries of individuals in the workplace with the goals of preserving lives, preventing further harm, and promoting recovery.

Figures 2 through 4 depict the 3 conceptual models of Stress First Aid for Healthcare Workers.[14] The *Stress Continuum* (see **Fig. 2**) serves as a dynamic lens for codifying self and others in relation to the presence of observable signs and symptoms of stress and their associated functional impairment. The value of a *stress continuum* lies in its ability to establish a shared mental model for stress in the workspace. In the *green zone*, one operates near their personal best with motivation to learn, grow, and excel. In the *yellow zone*, one is predictably reacting to stressful situations with the reasonable expectation of being able to return to our functional baseline without assistance. In the *orange zone,* one reacts more intensely to the *4 Sources of Orange Zone Stress* (**Fig. 3**) and finds it difficult to independently return to our functional

READY (Green)	REACTING (Yellow)	INJURED (Orange)	ILL (Red)
DEFINITION	**DEFINITION**	**DEFINITION**	**DEFINITION**
•Optimal functioning	•Mild and transient distress or impairment	•More severe and persistent distress or impairment	•Clinical mental disorder
•Adaptive growth	•Always goes away	•Leaves a scar	•Unhealed stress injury causing life impairment
•Wellness	•Low risk	•Higher risk	
FEATURES	**CAUSES**	**CAUSES**	**TYPES**
•At one's best	•Any stressor	•Life threat	•PTSD
•Well-trained and prepared	**FEATURES**	•Loss	•Depression
•In control	•Increased energy / HR	•Moral injury	•Anxiety
•Physically, mentally and spiritually fit	•Change in focus ↑↓	•Wear and tear	•Substance use disorders
•Mission-focused	•Feeling irritable, anxious	**FEATURES**	**FEATURES**
•Motivated	•Alert for threats	•Loss of control	•Symptoms persist and worsen over time
•Calm and steady	•Difficulty sleeping	•Panic, rage or depression	•Severe distress or social or occupational impairment
•Having fun	•Muscle tension or other physical changes	•No longer feeling like normal self	
•Behaving ethically		•Excessive guilt, shame or blame	
		•Misconduct	

Fig. 2. SFA doctrine: stress continuum. (Watson P, Westphal RJ. Stress First Aid for Health Care Workers. National Center for PTSD 2020. Available on: www.ptsd.va.gov.)

Trauma	Loss	Inner Conflict	Wear and Tear
A *traumatic* injury	A *grief* injury	A *moral* injury	A *fatigue* injury
Due to the experience of or exposure to intense injury, horrific or gruesome experiences, or death.	Due to the loss of people, things or parts of oneself.	Due to behaviors or the witnessing of behaviors that violate moral values.	Due to the accumulation of stress from all sources over time without sufficient rest and recovery.

Fig. 3. SFA doctrine: 4 sources of orange zone stress. (Watson P, Westphal RJ. Stress First Aid for Health Care Workers. National Center for PTSD 2020. Available on: www.ptsd.va.gov.)

baseline without prompt assistance. In the *red zone*, one is largely incapable of independently functioning and needs immediate assistance. One's relative position along the *stress continuum* is dynamic. That said, not every member of the community operates from a functional baseline in the *green zone*. An inherent value of the *stress continuum* lies in its ability to neutralize the impacts of mental illness stigma by normalizing and naming stress within the workspace. In this regard, Andy Andrews is right when he said, "We are all in a crisis, coming out of a crisis, or headed for a crisis."[25]

Zones of stress can be further characterized by their typical precipitants. Although *yellow zone stress* is defined by those ordinary life stressors unique to a particular situation or setting (eg, work schedule changes, traffic, and high nurse-to-patient ratios), *orange zone stress* is defined by those extraordinary forms of orange zone stress (eg, *trauma*, *loss*, *inner conflict*, and *wear and tear*) that strain our ability to independently cope (see **Fig. 3**). *Trauma* is an *orange zone stressor* defined by direct exposure to intense or protracted expressions of injury or death. *Loss* is an *orange zone stressor* defined by the loss of people, things, or aspects of oneself that fundamentally alter how one thinks, feels, and acts. *Inner conflict* is an *orange zone stressor* defined by exposure to morally distressing situations and circumstances that can transform one's sense of trust. Finally, *wear and tear* are *orange zone stressors* defined by the accumulation of both *yellow zone* and *orange zone* stresses in the presence of diminishing personal coping reserves. Individually and collectively, *orange zone stressors* confer a greater risk for both *orange zone* and *red zone* behaviors along the *stress continuum*. Reflecting on nursing's role during this pandemic, we would be hard-pressed to identify any nurse that has not been exposed to *orange zone stress*.

The *SFA* model (**Fig. 4**) is an alliterative algorithmic model designed to structure specific behaviors and actions in response to stress injury. Broken into 3 different categories (eg, *Continuous Aid*, *Primary Aid*, and *Secondary Aid*), there are 7 actions of the model. *Continuous aid* encompasses the *check* and *coordinate* actions. Reminiscent of the first elements of Basic Life Support,[26] the *Continuous aid* elements of *check* and *coordinate* require the individual to assess both self and environment for safety before engaging the peer in presumed distress. If the peer is found to be in *the red zone*, there is an indication to seek out immediate assistance within the formal health-care delivery system. As reflected in **Fig. 4**, the elements of *continuous aid* are ubiquitous through the SFA model. This suggests that one must remain vigilant to the potential for situations and circumstances to escalate necessitating referral.

SFA is less of a single intervention and more reflective of a sustained relationship. A peer trained in *SFA* uses the *stress continuum* as a prism from which they view peers in the workspace. When they encounter a peer in the *yellow*, *orange*, or *red zone* along the *stress continuum*, they act through *SFA*. If a peer is not perceived to be in immediate crisis (*red zone*), there is an indication to progress to *primary aid*. *Primary aid*, defined by *cover* and *calm*, is designed to promote a sense of physical and psychological safety, and calming. *Primary aid* behaviors can reflect efforts to remove a

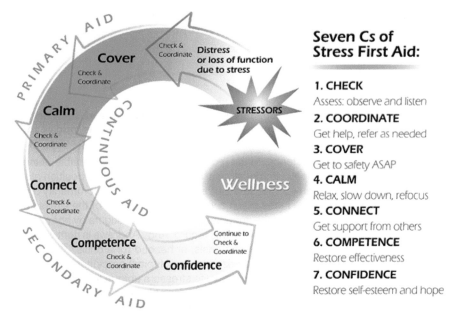

Seven Cs of Stress First Aid:

1. CHECK
Assess: observe and listen

2. COORDINATE
Get help, refer as needed

3. COVER
Get to safety ASAP

4. CALM
Relax, slow down, refocus

5. CONNECT
Get support from others

6. COMPETENCE
Restore effectiveness

7. CONFIDENCE
Restore self-esteem and hope

Fig. 4. SFA doctrine: SFA model. (Watson P, Westphal RJ. Stress First Aid for Health Care Workers. National Center for PTSD 2020. Available on: www.ptsd.va.gov.)

peer from a stressful situation, physically and emotionally protect a peer, and guide them through breathing or distraction exercises to reduce the negative impacts of acute stress. *Primary aid* behaviors are designed to help a peer experiencing stress calm their body and mind so that they are better able to think through (vs feel through) a stressful situation. *SFA* is not designed to be a resource that can be scheduled on a calendar.

Provided a peer is recovering and not actively in the *orange* or *red zone*, *secondary aid* is then indicated. Linking back to the core training objectives of *SFA*, if *continuous* and *primary aid* are designed to "preserve life" and "prevent further harm" *secondary aid* is designed to "promote recovery."[27] *Secondary aid* is composed of the *connect*, *competence*, and *confidence* actions. The *connect* action is designed to flood the peer with augmented social support to neutralize the sense of isolation that commonly occurs alongside a stress-related injury or illness. The *competence* action is designed to foster a renewed sense of personal, social, and professional competence because it is recognized that these can be lost in response to stress-related injury and illness. The *confidence* action is designed to help a peer experiencing stress to reestablish a personal sense of trust, hope, self-worth, and meaning.

STRESS FIRST AID EXEMPLAR
Stress First Aid for Healthcare Workers Pilot

The pressures placed on nursing programs during COVID-19 have been unprecedented. During the peak of the pandemic, the only academic sustainment options were to temporarily shut down programs or flip them online seemingly overnight. The rapid introduction of distance-based learning to ill-equipped programs illuminated weaknesses and vulnerabilities for both individuals and programs.[28] Martin and colleagues recognized that the COVID-19 pandemic significantly influenced students' preparedness and clinical competence yielding patient safety implications.[29]

Overbaugh and colleagues,[30] studied undergraduate nursing student's perceptions of the profession, stress, and coping during the pandemic. This study illuminated a relationship between stress and coping thematically focused on student transition to the nursing profession, educational barriers while in school, and challenges with faculty–student relationships.[30]

Coincidentally during the early stages of the COVID-19 pandemic, Duke University School of Nursing opened its Student Success Program (2020) designed to promote emotional health, provide academic support, and connect students to resources at Duke and beyond (Duke University School of Nursing, 2023). Funded by the Department of Health and Human Services Administration (HRSA) through a 109 Cooperative Agreement, Duke University partnered with North Carolina Central University to pilot Stress First Aid for Healthcare Workers training in support of its health profession's students (Health Resources & Services Administration, 2022). The SFA training offered on campus, virtual synchronous, hybrid on campus and virtual synchronous, and asynchronous recording delivery strategies to expedite student exposure to the training content. Duke University School of Nursing has adopted *Stress First Aid for Healthcare Workers* as a "Ticket to Matriculation" training requirement for all newly enrolled students and provides this training during initial program orientation.

The genesis of *Stress First Aid for Healthcare Workers* was born of seminal work within the Department of Navy.[13] During the pilot period, a cohort of faculty and staff with a particular interest in wellness initiatives was convened to help revise the content and delivery to align with the needs of an audience that included both busy clinicians and students. This group of 25 "champions" from Duke and NCCU underwent training and then divided into workgroups to review sessions and make recommendations with respect to (1) refinement of session content and format—particularly for online delivery, (2) design of application exercises and case studies, (3) engagement of stakeholders, and (4) identification of wellness resources. Based on champion recommendations, the content was streamlined, and the materials were adapted for both in-person and online delivery. Specific qualitative changes were also made to the training content to reduce the military-centric language and foster diversity, equity, and inclusion.

As established (**Fig. 5**), the initial training content introduced the foundational elements of SFA (eg, Stress Continuum, 4 Sources of Orange Zone Stress, and the Stress First Aid model) and was 4 hours in length. Subsequent 1-hour long virtual booster sessions were scheduled monthly to apply SFA principles in relation to high volume, high risk, and problem-prone scenarios commonly seen within health professions education.

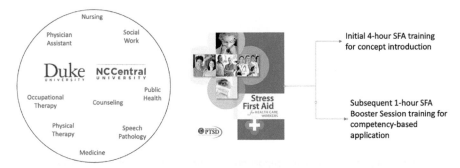

Fig. 5. Duke & North Carolina University pilot for SFA for the health-care worker.

PROGRAM EVALUATION

During the pilot, we continued to offer in-person and synchronous virtual training to audiences of faculty, staff, and students at our institutions and others across the state. Evaluation metrics for these sessions included simple demographics with the number attending by institution and profession. Beginning in July 2022, attendees were also asked to respond to a short feedback survey and a 3-item knowledge assessment. Continuing education credits were available on request. The proposal for SFA training was reviewed by the Instituational Review Board (IRB) and determined to be exempt as nonresearch.

In a 12-month period between July 2022 and June 2023, 15 SFA training sessions were conducted that reached 905 participants. Of these, 3 sessions were exclusively virtual via Zoom, one was hybrid, and all others were in-person. Three sessions targeted matriculating nursing students from Duke University including 128 total students in the Accelerated Bachelor of Science of Nursing program, 241 in Advance Practice Nursing degree tracks (Master of Science in Nursing [MSN], Doctor of Nursing Practice [DNP], and Certified Registered Nurse Anesthetist [CRNA]), and 50 on a post-Masters/PhD track. Among 13 remaining sessions, 8 were offered at Duke, 3 at North Carolina Central University (NCCU), and 1 each at Fayetteville State and UNC-Chapel Hill. **Figure 6** provides a breakdown of the self-reported profession of 516 (57%) attendees responding to online surveys from across these different sessions. Among 514 participants taking the 3-item knowledge assessment, 309 (60.1%) answered all questions correctly and 188 (36.6%) got 2 of 3 questions right. Participants rated the training positively across all domains on the feedback survey (see **Fig. 6**). Qualitative content analysis of open-ended responses revealed a high level of satisfaction with the course content and the facilitators (**Table 1**). Some attendees suggested providing additional resources (eg, handouts or slides) to reinforce learning and adding or enhancing sessions focused on the application of SFA principles with practice scenarios and role plays. In response to this last point, 3 one-hour virtual booster sessions were piloted that included 19 participants.

In the coming year, plans are underway to launch our online content via the open online course provider, Coursera. Participants will have access to video recordings and

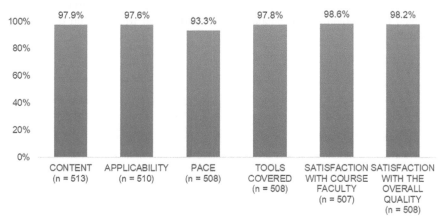

Fig. 6. Percentage of respondents reporting "satisfied/very satisfied" for SFA evaluation items.

Table 1
Stress first aid table

	Continuous Aid Behaviors
Check	• Assess personal capacity to effectively leverage SFA principles before engaging a stress injured peer in the workspace • Assess stress-injured peer in relation to both the stress continuum and the 4 sources of orange zone stress • Assess all members of the health-care team in relation to both the stress continuum and the 4 sources of orange zone stress • Assess environment of care for modifiable sources of stress and seek out support from leadership to enact change
Coordinate	• Connect peers demonstrating red zone behavior with immediate formal support • Connect peers that seem to be reacting to stress with yellow and orange zone behavior to available resources for stress reduction • Communicate deidentified stress-related themes and patterns to leadership for action • Seek out personal assistance if the SFA support offered to others begins to manifest as a stress injury
Primary aid behaviors	
Cover	• Ensure personal safety ahead of engaging peer with SFA • Take action to ensure safety of stress-injured peer • Take action to protect all in the workspace from harm and injury • Take action to reduce chaos in the workspace
Calm	• Engage stress-injured peer with a calm and reassuring demeanor • Lead stress-injured peer in calming techniques • Empathically engage peer, leveraging active listening skills and using unconditional positive regard • Use centering techniques to maintain stress injured peer's attention
Secondary aid behaviors	
Connect	• Take action to personally connect with stress-injured peer through multiple means and mediums • Seek out opportunities to augment social support system for stress-injured peer in the workspace • Facilitate increased communication between the stress-injured peer and other members of the team • Roll with resistance if stress-injured peer rebuffs your attempts to connect
Competence	• Encourage a progressive return to independent occupational functioning • Seek out opportunities to have stress-injured peer perform that which they are both comfortable with and enjoy doing early • Offer repeated assistance and recognize success • Validate evidence of competence both privately and publicly
Confidence	• Earn a stress-injured peer's trust through reliable engagement

(continued on next page)

Table 1 (continued)	
	Continuous Aid Behaviors
	• Recognize that orange zone stress has potentially degraded the stress-injured peer's sense of hope and self-worth, which will take time to remobilize
• Project confidence in the stress-injured peer's capacity and abilities publicly
• Highlight what is working well in the occupational space and deemphasize what is not

Pat is a registered nurse working in critical care for the past 3 y. Pat graduated from nursing school in 2020 and was hired 2 mo before COVID-19 began to dominate the hospital setting. Similar to other members of the health-care team, Pat was exposed to much orange zone stress (eg, trauma, loss, inner conflict, and wear and tear) during the pandemic. Pat contracted COVID-19 twice during this time. Pat has been vacillating between the yellow and orange zone for the past 3 y. Earlier this year, Pat's coping reserves depleted pushing Pat into the red zone, which led to a suicide attempt and a subsequent 2-wk psychiatric hospitalization. Following the hospitalization, Pat has been on FMLA participating in intensive outpatient psychiatric care. Although better, Pat is not yet well. Pat is planning on returning to work next month. In anticipation of returning, Pat communicated with both the nursing supervisor as well as some trusted peers at work. The below table reflects strategies to apply SFA principles dynamically during Pat's recovery. FMLA, Family Medical Leave Act.

discussion boards. They will also have the option of enrolling in synchronous online booster sessions to practice applying the principles of SFA in a case-based format. The flexibility of the online course will allow the team to reach many more students, staff, and faculty in various locations with disparate schedules. Of course, in-person training sessions will continue to be offered as demand warrants. Plans are underway to adapt the evaluation to include measures of self-efficacy (adapted from the Wisdom and Well-being Peer Support Training program at the University of Virginia, School of Nursing) and baseline measures of emotional exhaustion and work–life balance.

SUMMARY

Although the framework[13,14,16] that informs SFA has been in place for years, widespread implementation in health-care delivery systems and health professions education is in its early stages. Developed by the federal government, *Stress First Aid for Healthcare Workers* is a free resource that has been effectively applied within the Department of Defense, Department of Veteran Affairs, National Guard units, first responder units, health centers, and academic systems across the nation. Although health-care management aims to mitigate unnecessary and modifiable stress(ors) in the workspace, it is unrealistic to expect a stress-free workspace. Alternatively, embracing a framework like *Stress First Aid for Healthcare Worke*rs creates an opportunity to mobilize peer support to recognize and reduce the impact of occupational stress in the workspace with the goals of *preserving life, preventing further harm,* and *promoting recovery. Stress First Aid for Healthcare Workers* offers a new language around stress that can support health promotion, illness prevention, and stigma reduction. This review describes the successful implementation of *SFA* for faculty, clinicians, students, and staff across multiple institutions with a flexible approach combining in-person and online training and application sessions. Ultimately, such a multipronged approach aimed at the current and future health professionals has the greatest promise for achieving a lasting reduction in occupational stress in health care.

CLINICS CARE POINTS

- Post-COVID-19, *orange zone stress* (eg, trauma, loss, inner conflict, and wear and tear) has complicated traditional occupational stressors for nurses (eg, rotating shifts, nurse-to-patient ratios, and interprofessional and intraprofessional conflicts) increasing vulnerability to stress and stress-related injuries.
- Occupational stress management in health care is best when systematically and proactively performed in equal partnership between employer and employee.
- The health-care delivery system illustrates a positive bias toward those symptoms and stressors that exist at or above a clinical threshold of significance. This is particularly so when it comes to stress-related injury and illness.
- The stress continuum serves as a shared mental model to operationalize occupational stress intent to recognize and respond to stress injury earlier.

DISCLOSURE

Support for the program, from which this article evolves, came from the HRSA through a 109 Cooperative Agreement (Award Number: 1 U3NHP45396-01-00) funded by the American Rescue Plan Act of 2021 P L. 117 to 2, Section 2703 42 U.S C. § 295.

REFERENCES

1. Mental Health America. The Mental Health of Healthcare Workers in COVID-19. Mental Health America Funded by Johnson & Johnson Foundation. https://mhanational.org/mental-health-healthcare-workers-covid-19. Accessed April 27, 2023, 2023.
2. Riedel B, Horen SR, Reynolds A, et al. Mental health disorders in nurses during the COVID-19 pandemic: implications and coping strategies. Front Public Health 2021;9:707358.
3. AMN Healthcare. Survey of 18,000 Nurses Shows Worsening Satisfaction and Wellbeing. 2023. https://www.amnhealthcare.com/amn-insights/nursing/surveys/2023/
4. Dyrbye LN, West CP, Satele D, et al. Burnout among U.S. medical students, residents, and early career physicians relative to the general U.S. population. Acad Med : Journal of the Association Of American Medical Colleges 2014;89(3): 443–51.
5. Goebert D, Thompson D, Takeshita J, et al. Depressive symptoms in medical students and residents: a multischool study. Acad Med : Journal of the Association Of American Medical Colleges 2009;84(2):236–41.
6. Feaster B, McKinley-Grant L, McMichael AJ. Microaggressions in medicine. Cutis 2021;107(5):235–7.
7. Luberto CM, Goodman JH, Halvorson B, et al. Stress and Coping Among Health Professions Students During COVID-19: A Perspective on the Benefits of Mindfulness. Glob Adv Health Med 2020;9. https://doi.org/10.1177/2164956120977827. 2164956120977827.
8. Kelsey EA, West CP, Cipriano PF, et al. Original research: suicidal ideation and attitudes toward help seeking in U.S. nurses relative to the general working population. Am J Nurs 2021;121(11):24–36.

9. Centers for Disease Control and Prevention. (1999). *Stress... At Work.* Washington DC: Centers for Disease Control and Prevention. Available at: https://www.cdc.gov/niosh/docs/99-101/default.html.

10. Reducing risks for mental disorders: frontiers for preventive intervention research. The National Academies Press.; 1994.

11. American Psychiatric Association. Diagnostic and statistical manual of mental disorders : DSM-5. 5th edition. American Psychiatric Association; 2013. p. 947.

12. Koenen KC, Ratanatharathorn A, Ng L, et al. Posttraumatic stress disorder in the World Mental Health Surveys. Psychol Med 2017;47(13):2260–74.

13. Nash W.P., Westphal R.J., Watson P., Litz B.T., *Combat and Operational Stress First-Aid (COSFA) Training Manual.* Washington, DC, 2010. Available at: http://www.alsbom-gm.org/files/COSFA%20NAVY%20TM.pdf.

14. Stress first aid for health care workers (U. S. Department of Veterans Affairs) 97 (2021).

15. Hobfoll SE, Watson P, Bell CC, et al. Five essential elements of immediate and mid-term mass trauma intervention: empirical evidence. Psychiatry. Winter 2007;70(4):283–315, discussion 316-69.

16. Hobfoll SE, Watson P, Bell CC, et al. Five essential elements of immediate and mid-term mass trauma intervention: empirical evidence. Psychiatry. Winter 2021;84(4):311–46.

17. Corey J, Vallieres F, Frawley T, et al. A rapid realist review of group psychological first aid for humanitarian workers and volunteers. Int J Environ Res Publ Health 2021;18(4). https://doi.org/10.3390/ijerph18041452.

18. Kilic N, Simsek N. The effects of psychological first aid training on disaster preparedness perception and self-efficacy. Nurse Educ Today 2019;83:104203.

19. Schultz PP, Ryan RM, Niemiec CP, et al. Mindfulness, work climate, and psychological need satisfaction in employee well-being. Mindfulness 2015;6(5):971–85.

20. Watson P, Taylor V, Gist R, et al. Stress First Aid for Firefighters and Emergency Medical Services Personnel. 2015.

21. Malik M, Peirce J, Wert MV, et al. Psychological first aid well-being support rounds for frontline healthcare workers during COVID-19. Front Psychiatr 2021; 12:669009.

22. Kantaris X, Radcliffe M, Acott K, et al. Training healthcare assistants working in adult acute inpatient wards in Psychological First Aid: An implementation and evaluation study. J Psychiatr Ment Health Nurs 2020;27(6):742–51.

23. Blake H, Mahmood I, Dushi G, et al. Psychological impacts of COVID-19 on healthcare trainees and perceptions towards a digital wellbeing support package. Int J Environ Res Publ Health 2021;18(20). https://doi.org/10.3390/ijerph182010647.

24. Kameno Y, Hanada A, Asai D, et al. Individual psychotherapy using psychological first aid for frontline nurses at high risk of psychological distress during the COVID-19 pandemic. Psychiatr Clin Neurosci 2021;75(1):25–7.

25. Andrews A. The noticer returns : sometimes you find perspective, and sometimes perspective finds you. W Pub. Group, an imprint of Thomas Nelson; 2013. p. 227.

26. Hazinski MF, American Heart Association. Basic life support : provider manual, ix. American Heart Association; 2016. p. 85.

27. Stress First Aid for Health Care Professionals, Recognize and Respond Early to Stress Injuries.

28. Kartsoni E, Bakalis N, Markakis G, et al. Distance learning in nursing education during the COVID-19 pandemic: psychosocial impact for the greek nursing

students-a qualitative approach. Healthcare (Basel) 2023;11(8). https://doi.org/10.3390/healthcare11081178.

29. Martin B, Kaminski-Ozturk N, Smiley R, et al. Assessing the impact of the COVID-19 pandemic on nursing education: a national study of prelicensure RN programs. J Nurs Regul 2023;14(1):S1–67.

30. Overbaugh KJ, Monforto K, DiGiacomo P, et al. Understanding COVID-19's impact on nursing students' education, professional perceptions, stress, and coping. Nurs Educ Perspect 2022;43(6):E47–9.

Opportunities for Nurses to Decrease the Stigma Associated with Housing Instability and Homelessness

Donna J. Biederman, DrPH, MN, RN, CPH[a],*,
Heather O'Donohue, MS, BSN, RN[b], Julia Gamble, MSN, NP[c]

KEYWORDS

- Homelessness • Housing instability • Stigma • ICD-10-CM • Medical respite
- Policy • Interventions • Socio-ecological model

KEY POINTS

- People experiencing homelessness (PEH) and housing instability frequently encounter stigma.
- PEH and housing instability often have multiple health conditions and are less well than people who are housed.
- The stigma surrounding housing instability can lead to health disparities.
- The socioecological model illustrates opportunities for nurse intervention to decrease stigma and increase health outcomes for PEH and housing instability.

INTRODUCTION

In the past 5 years, the number of people experiencing homelessness (PEH) in the United States has increased.[1] PEH have a higher disease burden (eg, chronic illness, mental illness, substance use disorder [SUD]) and early mortality compared to people who are housed.[2] Stigma adds to the burden of disease and disease management for PEH.[3] In this article the authors (1) review stigma, (2) define housing and homelessness, (3) describe the health and health care disparities PEH experience, and (4) using the socio-ecological model as a framework, offer opportunities for nurses to intervene in efforts to decrease the stigma that PEH and housing instability encounter to improve health outcomes.

---

[a] Duke University School of Nursing, DUMC 3322, 307 Trent Drive, Durham, NC 27710, USA;
[b] New Hanover Regional Medical Center, 2131 South 17th Street, Wilmington, NC 28403, USA;
[c] Duke Outpatient Clinic, 4220 North Roxboro Street, 2nd Floor, Durham, NC 27704, USA
* Corresponding author.
E-mail address: Donna.biederman@duke.edu

Nurs Clin N Am 59 (2024) 63–74
https://doi.org/10.1016/j.cnur.2023.11.013
nursing.theclinics.com
0029-6465/24/© 2023 Elsevier Inc. All rights reserved.

Stigma

In his seminal work, *Stigma: Notes on the Management of Spoiled Identity*, Erving Goffman[4] described stigma as a discrepancy between individual attributes and socially created norms that results in an individual being "discredited" by society. A group convened by the National Academies of Sciences, Engineering, and Medicine described 3 types of stigmas.[5] Some such attributes are observable but some are not necessarily obvious. Sociologists have described a dynamic at work in the stigma that results in a power imbalance.[6] This dynamic starts with labeling an individual or group as "other" and describing that group as inherently different and of less value. This can have an impact on the individual's sense of self (self-stigma) and the perception of others toward that person (public stigma). The end result can be a reduction in access to resources (structural stigma) and an increase in stress which can lead to worsening overall health[6,7] (**Table 1**). Lack of housing has been shown to be a source of stigma.[3]

DEFINITIONS
Housing

The World Health Organization defines housing as a social determinant of health (SDOH)—a nonmedical factor that influences health outcomes.[8] The US Department of Health and Human Services (DHHS) has included housing concerns in Healthy People 2030, the national health goals for the United States.[9] Clinicians who work with PEH affirm that "housing is health care"[10] as a home provides a location to safely store medications, a location to access in-home services such as home health or hospice, and a pickup location for transportation to appointments. A home also provides a location for rest, nourishment, and hygiene.

Homelessness

In the United States, the federal government funds shelters, housing, health, and education services for PEH. Unfortunately, various federal departments have different definitions for homelessness. The US Department of Housing and Urban Development (HUD) is the primary funder of homeless services and has four categories that include housing instability and homelessness[11] (**Table 2**).

Table 1 Types of stigmas[5]	
Type of Stigmas	**Definition**
Self-stigma	Individual internalization and acceptance of negative stereotypes resulting in an individual feeling "broken".
Public stigma (or social stigma)	Society's negative attitude toward a particular group of people with a stigmatized condition resulting in an environment in which people with such conditions are discredited, feared, and isolated.
Structural stigma	System-level discrimination (eg, cultural norms, institutional practices, health care policies not at parity with other health conditions) resulting in constrained resources and opportunities impairing well-being.

Adapted from Committee on the Science of Changing Behavioral Health Social Norms, Board on Behavioral, Cognitive, and Sensory Sciences, Division of Behavioral and Social Sciences and Education, National Academies of Sciences, Engineering, and Medicine. Ending Discrimination Against People with Mental and Substance Use Disorders: The Evidence for Stigma Change. National Academies Press (US); 2016. Accessed September 18, 2023. http://www.ncbi.nlm.nih.gov/books/NBK384915/

Table 2
Homeless categories—US Department of Housing and Urban Development definitions[11]

Category 1 Literally homeless	• Persons living somewhere that is "not fit for human habitation" (eg, car, abandoned building, tent) • Persons living in a shelter or in a transitional or hotel setting funded by a charitable organization (like churches/homeless service providers) • Persons who were in an institution (eg, jail, hospital) for the past 90 days and was in a shelter or on streets prior to that
Category 2 Imminent risk of homelessness	Persons who will lose housing they own, rent, or reside in within 14 days and have no identified location to go to after this
Category 3 Unaccompanied youth under 25	Persons who do not meet Category 1 or 2 criteria may meet Category 3 criteria if they have not had housing for 60 days
Category 4 Domestic violence	Persons fleeing or attempting to flee domestic violence who have no other location to go

Adapted from HUD. Four Categories in the Homeless Definition. Published 2023. Accessed September 18, 2023. https://www.hudexchange.info/homelessness-assistance/coc-esg-virtual-binders/coc-esg-homeless-eligibility/four-categories

The US Department of Education and the DHHS include the HUD categories as well as people who are living in unstable housing situations such as adults living with family, "couch surfing" with acquaintances, or paying for expensive motel rooms.

PEH advocates are concerned that the numbers used to quantify PEH are artificially low as they do not fully capture the number of people experiencing housing instability and the "hidden homelessness" due to the focus on the narrow HUD categories in community counts of PEH.[12] For example, 2019 HUD data indicated that there were approximately 570,000 PEH. When the HUD definition of homelessness is expanded to include those who are "doubled-up" (which is included in the US Department of Education's homelessness definition), the number of PEH in 2019 expands exponentially to 3.7 million.[13] This has an impact on local, state, and federal planning for housing support including funding new construction of affordable housing, funding rental supports for existing housing, and funding services such as shelters or case managers.

DISCUSSION
Housing Instability, Homelessness, and Health

PEH have high rates of chronic illness.[2] Often times, chronic illness is accompanied by SUD and mental illness—a condition known as trimorbidity.[14,15] PEH also have higher rates of death—commonly referred to as "premature mortality"—earlier than expected based on age as compared to people in housing.[2] This increased mortality persists when chronically homeless people are housed.[16]

PEH frequently delay seeking care[17] for a variety of reasons including prioritizing basic needs such as safe shelter and food, lack of insurance or payment, and transportation. Oftentimes, PEH have multiple issues that demand attention occurring in multiple social domains.[18] Stigma is an additional factor that impacts the health and health care of PEH and housing instability. For instance, women living with human immunodeficiency virus (HIV) described how the lack of privacy in congregate housing resulted in decreased medication adherence and provider appointment attendance for fear of HIV status disclosure. Comorbidities, including physical and mental health issues, SUD, and food insecurity, also affected their ability to adhere to their HIV medication regimens. Through it all, the overlapping stigma of all of these issues impacted them negatively.[19]

Housing Instability, Homelessness, and Health Disparities

Housing instability and homelessness contribute to health disparities. Research in health areas such as cardiac disease, cancer, pregnancy, and infectious diseases has found that PEH experience higher levels of mortality and are less likely to receive specialized services.[20] PEH are more likely to die from complications of cardiovascular disease (eg, myocardial infarction, stroke) and less likely to receive procedural interventions.[20] Cancer care and outcomes are also negatively impacted by homelessness and housing instability.[21] Housing instability increases risks for poor pregnancy outcomes including low birth weight and prematurity.[22] Housing difficulties have been associated with an increased self-stigma in PEH regarding having HIV as compared to HIV-positive people who are housed.[23] The coronavirus disease 2019 (COVID-19) pandemic had a significant impact on PEH and exacerbated housing instability as financial insecurity led to evictions and homelessness. Housing displacement and overcrowding had a direct impact on increased COVID-19 infections among already vulnerable populations.[24–26]

Stigma, the Socio-Ecological Model, and Opportunities for Nursing Intervention

Stigma represents the attitudes, beliefs, behaviors, and structures that interact at different levels of society (ie, individuals, groups, organizations, systems). It manifests in prejudicial attitudes and discriminatory practices against PEH, producing adverse health outcomes. The social-ecological perspective empowers clinicians and researchers to create and implement interventions ameliorating the stigma of homelessness in health care settings at multiple levels of analysis.[27] It reveals homelessness is due to contextual factors that interact with vulnerabilities impacted by social, cultural, structural, and personal influences. There are many examples of stigma in health care.[28] Valdez noted that the use of stigmatizing language and labeling of patients perpetuates harmful stereotypes and biases and the label 'homeless' in medical documentation dehumanizes individuals and implies they are unworthy of care. Other studies have found that stigma in health facilities can lead to denial of care, inferior care, and physical and verbal abuse.[3,29–31] Despite unequivocal scientific evidence on the prevalence of stigma in health care facilities and its impact on the well-being of PEH, few interventions are implemented.

The ecological systems theory developed by Bronfenbrenner (1977)[32] is a theoretic framework for understanding how distinct levels of the environment interact to create the phenotype of an individual. The original theory by Bronfenbrenner illustrated nesting spheres that place the individual in the center encompassed by various systems of influence. McLeroy and colleagues[27] adapted the socio-ecological model to create interventions for health-related problems and include the levels of individual, interpersonal, organizational, community, and policy. The model is typically still represented by concentric circles; however, the levels of influence have changed (**Fig. 1**).

The 5 nested spheres of the socio-ecological model illustrate different levels of influence on individual behavior. This model is often used to develop interventions to improve health behaviors and outcomes. Most often, those interventions are focused on clients, patients, or community members. However, the model can be used to illustrate how clinicians can intervene to make changes along the spectrum of influences that can affect individual and population health. In the remainder of this section, the

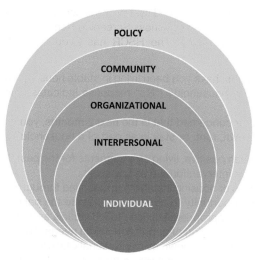

Fig. 1. Socio-ecological model.

authors present interventions at each level of the model that nurses could employ to decrease the stigma surrounding PEH and housing instability.

Individual Level

The individual level identifies personal factors that lead to the stigma of PEH. Interventions focus on the beliefs, biases, and attitudes of health care practitioners. Anecdotal reports from PEH emphasize staff attitudes as essential in successful care.[33,34] Holding oneself accountable regarding labels used to describe PEH in the clinical setting can reduce language that alienates PEH and biases other health care practitioners.[28,35]

Interpersonal Level

The interpersonal level aims to influence the behaviors within social relationships that create and perpetuate stigma, thus altering social norms and culture over time. Interpersonal interventions include education on both stigma and homelessness and open dialog regarding ways to eliminate practitioner bias in our interactions with homeless patients. Peer advocates who have personal experience with housing instability can assist in reducing stigma through coaching health care workers in their language use and communication techniques. Peer advocates can also work as part of the health care team to assist patients in identifying solutions and providing support. The shared experience and role modeling of the peer advocate can improve life skills and health outcomes including reducing substance use for patients with SUD.[36,37]

Organizational Level

Screening for housing instability in health care settings is a recommended best practice and, as of 2023, is required for Joint Commission accredited entities.[38] However, implementation of screening in health care settings is variable. A 2019 study demonstrated that of more than 700 US hospitals, less than 25% did comprehensive SDOHs screening and 33% did no SDOHs screening.[39] Screening was more likely to occur when mandated by insurance companies (state Medicaid or private-managed care organizations) or government funding (such as community health centers).[39] In 2012, the

Veteran's Administration implemented system-wide screening for homelessness. The screening tool is called the Homelessness Screening Reminder (HSCR) and is part of the electronic medical record.[40] The HSCR has 2 questions to assess housing instability:

1. "In the past 2 months, have you been living in stable housing that you own, rent, or stay in as part of a household? ("No" response indicates veteran is positive for homelessness.)"
2. "Are you worried or concerned that in the next 2 months, you may **not** have stable housing that you own, rent, or stay in as part of a household?"

For those who screen positive, living arrangements for the past 2 months and desirability of a social work intervention are assessed.[40]

When homelessness or housing instability is identified through screening in a health care setting, it is an opportunity to add this problem to the patient's diagnosis list to provide resources and appropriate services to individuals as well as to create opportunities for better understanding of population health needs. The codes that are associated with medical billing are known as International Classification of Diseases, Tenth Revision (ICD-10) codes and they include codes that are relevant to housing and other social needs (**Table 3**). Please note this is just a sampling of the ICD-10 "Z" codes related to SDOHs. For a more comprehensive list, please see the CDC ICD-10 CM site at https://icd10cmtool.cdc.gov/?fy=FY2023.

The federal Centers for Medicare and Medicaid Services and a consortium of health care entities including the American Hospital Association have approved guidelines regarding the use of ICD-10 codes. These organizations have published recommendations indicating that for ICD-10 codes related to social needs (such as housing), it is possible for nursing (or other health care providers who are not explicitly billing as the patient's medical provider) to document these codes in the medical record if it is allowed by their employer.[41,42] A useful infographic for ICD-10 Clinical Modification (ICD-10-CM) code use along the health care spectrum is available on the following uniform resource locator: https://www.cms.gov/files/document/zcodes-infographic.pdf.

Identifying housing instability and homelessness is important for safe patient care. Lack of awareness of a patient's housing situation can result in unsafe hospital discharges, inadequate care, or unrealistic medication regimens.[43] In a mixed-methods study of PEH who had been discharged from a hospital, more than half were not asked about their housing status.[44] Those who were asked about homelessness received resources for accessing needed health-related services (eg, transportation, medications, follow-up care).[44] Interestingly, qualitative analyses revealed a reluctance to discuss housing status related to stigma.[44]

Table 3
International Classification of Diseases, Tenth Revision codes relevant to housing instability and other social determinants of health

Z59.0	Homelessness
Z59.1	Inadequate housing
Z59.4	Lack of adequate food
Z91.120	Intentional underdosing of medication due to financial hardship
Z59.82	Transportation insecurity

If a health care system has processes to assess and document housing status, people who screen positive can be prioritized for testing or treatment prior to discharge (for example, rather than returning for outpatient colonoscopy to workup unexplained anemia and hematochezia, a patient may be assisted with an inpatient colonoscopy prep and procedure). Medications can be ordered that do not require refrigeration or multiple doses a day both of which can be difficult for people experiencing housing instability. Discharge planners can work with community services to identify locations that can accommodate home health visits to provide appropriate wound care, administration of intravenous antibiotics, or provision of home health physical therapy. All of these options require the identification of homelessness as a starting point. Nurses working in any setting can be a part of that process.

Community Level

PEH with medical problems may not be able to safely live on the street or in shelters following hospitalization due to a need for specialized services or recovery time. In some instances, they may be safe in their current setting but cannot access needed services due to an inability to prepare for a test (such as a colonoscopy which requires a 2-day preparation) or recover from a procedure (eg, cataract surgery). Also, it is important to note that housing instability and homelessness can be a result of hospitalization. Medical respite is the term used to describe short-term, nonhospital locations that can help PEH have a place to heal and access medical and supportive services.[45] Medical respite programs serve many functions and bridge the structural stigma imposed by some systems, including some health care institutions. Most medical respite settings develop because of a perceived need by health care systems or community homeless service providers or both. Medical respite settings vary in size, service model, and funding source. In 2023, there were 151 medical respite programs listed in the National Health Care for the Homeless Council's Medical Respite Care Directory.[46]

The reduction of hospital bed days and the provision of safe discharge options for hospitals are the impetus for medical respite programs in many communities. Most medical respite programs prioritize connecting PEH with access to ongoing support agencies and services. The authors' team led efforts to develop and implement a medical respite program in Durham, North Carolina. This work was a grassroots initiative that began in the community. The program, Durham Homeless Care Transitions (DHCT) is administered through Project Access of Durham County; a community-based organization. With DHCT, increased outpatient visits,[47] decreased emergency department visits,[48] and decreased hospital admissions have been seen.[47,48] Programmatic outcomes (eg, increased access to transportation; improved housing arrangement) were similar for PEH with and without diagnosed SUD,[48] a stigmatized medical condition. Sometimes the medical respite is a place to receive palliative services and a peaceful death. Hospice services are not available on the streets and PEH or housing instability need a place to die with dignity.[49] The exemplar in the following section demonstrates the authors' experience in 1 such case.

Exemplar

A 59-year-old man was referred to the authors' program by a local academic medical center. The hospital was about to discharge him when they realized he had nowhere to go. Prior to coming to the hospital, he had lived under a highway overpass, for 6 years, after losing his housing to a fire. He had no income other than panhandling, no health insurance, no primary care, and no housing. He had arrived at the hospital unable to walk as a result of pronounced nutritional deficiency. Over the course of his hospital stay, he was given vitamin B12 and regained his ability to walk. During his admission, he was diagnosed with a lung nodule thought to be an early lung cancer secondary to a lifetime of tobacco use. The authors worked to engage him and assist him in navigating connections to important resources including benefits (income/insurance), housing (with rent/utilities covered), and connection to medical and specialty care. He was linked to an intensive mental health community team and psychiatrist. Ultimately, when his lung cancer progressed, he was able to receive hospice services in his home where he died peacefully.

Policy Level

Federal, state, and local laws and regulations direct health care practice and related funding. Discriminatory policies, laws, and regulations endorse stigma on the individual level and are thus a necessary intervention for reducing stigma. Policy dictates how homelessness is defined and policymakers determine eligibility for resources. Laws in every state criminalize and ostracize PEH, preventing access to adequate health care and perpetuating stigma.[50] Nurses must be aware of policies that affect their patients at all levels of government.

For example, the Housing First program helps to eliminate barriers for PEH and housing instability who may be more difficult to house due to SUD and/or mental health problems. HUD champions evidence-based solutions to eliminate barriers to housing by endorsing the Housing First program. Housing First provides housing for PEH in addition to voluntary services that promote success in the community. New legislation introduced as the Housing Plus Act threatens the success of Housing First by diverting funding to programs that create barriers to housing PEH.[51] Nurses can intervene by becoming active in organizations that lobby Congress and influence political decision-making. Even membership in a professional organization helps with this cause. Nurses may also aspire to be policymakers to introduce and support policy efforts that decrease stigma through decreasing bias and discrimination in social and health care policies.

SUMMARY

PEH and housing insecurity frequently encounter self, public, and structural stigma. Nurses are well positioned to decrease stigma through developing, implementing, and/or supporting evidence-based interventions. The socio-ecological model serves as a guide to target interventions among multiple levels of influence. Nurses can work at any, multiple, or all levels of the socio-ecological model to make changes and assist in creating a more just and bias-free society.

CLINICS CARE POINTS

- Documenting housing status, and other SDOHs, is paramount to adequate patient care. This may be a first step in increasing dialog about housing instability and may help decrease associated stigma. ICD-10-CM codes are the best way to document housing status as they are easily searchable in the medical record and populate the patient's problem list. Clinicians, including registered nurses, can use ICD-10-CM codes when supported by organizational policy.

- Medical respite programs are beneficial to health care systems and PEH. Nurses, at all levels, should increase their knowledge of these programs and advocate (and participate in program development) if a medical respite is not available in their area.

- Nurses can influence policies, at multiple levels, in multiple ways. Supporting a professional organization that advocates for housing and other policy change that affects PEH and housing instability is helpful. The National Health Care for the Homeless Council (https://nhchc.org/) is one such organization.

DISCLOSURE

The authors have nothing to disclose.

REFERENCES

1. National alliance to end homelessness. State of homelessness: 2023 edition. National Alliance to End Homelessness; 2023. Available at: https://endhomelessness.org/homelessness-in-america/homelessness-statistics/state-of-homelessness/. Accessed September 15, 2023.
2. Fazel S, Geddes JR, Kushel M. The health of homeless people in high-income countries: descriptive epidemiology, health consequences, and clinical and policy recommendations. Lancet 2014;384(9953):1529–40. https://doi.org/10.1016/S0140-6736(14)61132-6.
3. Reilly J, Ho I, Williamson A. A systematic review of the effect of stigma on the health of people experiencing homelessness. Health Soc Care Community 2022;30(6): 2128–41. https://doi.org/10.1111/hsc.13884.
4. Goffman E. Stigma: Notes on the management of spoiled identity. New York, NY: Touchstone; 1963.
5. Committee on the Science of Changing Behavioral Health Social Norms, Board on Behavioral, Cognitive, and Sensory Sciences, Division of Behavioral and Social Sciences and Education, National Academies of Sciences, Engineering, and Medicine. Ending discrimination against people with mental and substance use disorders: the evidence for stigma change. National Academies Press (US); 2016. Available at: http://www.ncbi.nlm.nih.gov/books/NBK384915/. Accessed September 18, 2023.
6. Link BG, Phelan JC. Conceptualizing Stigma. Annu Rev Sociol 2001;27(1): 363–85. https://doi.org/10.1146/annurev.soc.27.1.363.
7. Hatzenbuehler ML, Phelan JC, Link BG. Stigma as a fundamental cause of population health inequalities. Am J Publ Health 2013;103(5):813–21.
8. World Health Organization. Social determinants of health. Published 2023. Available at: https://www.who.int/health-topics/social-determinants-of-health. Accessed September 14, 2023.
9. US DHHS. Social Determinants of Health - Healthy People 2030 | health.gov. Available at: https://health.gov/healthypeople/priority-areas/social-determinants-health. Accessed September 14, 2023.
10. Lozier J. Housing-is-Health-Care. Published n.d. https://nhchc.org/wp-content/uploads/2019/08/Housing-is-Health-Care.pdf. Accessed September 14, 2023.
11. HUD. Four Categories in the Homeless Definition. Published 2023. Available at: https://www.hudexchange.info/homelessness-assistance/coc-esg-virtual-binders/coc-esg-homeless-eligibility/four-categories. Accessed September 18, 2023.
12. Chicago Coalition for the Homeless. Hidden Homelessness in the United States. Chicago Coalition for the Homeless. Published March 3, 2023. https://www.chicagohomeless.org/hidden-homelessness-in-the-united-states/. Accessed September 13, 2023.

13. Richard MK, Dworkin J, Rule KG, et al. Quantifying Doubled-Up Homelessness: Presenting a New Measure Using U.S. Census Microdata. Housing Policy Debate 2022;0(0):1–22. https://doi.org/10.1080/10511482.2021.1981976.

14. Smith CM, Feigal J, Sloane R, et al. Differences in clinical outcomes of adults referred to a homeless transitional care program based on multimorbid health profiles: a latent class analysis. Front Psychiatr 2021;12. Available at: https://www.frontiersin.org/articles/10.3389/fpsyt.2021.780366. Accessed September 13, 2023.

15. Vickery KD, Winkelman TNA, Ford BR, et al. Trends in trimorbidity among adults experiencing homelessness in Minnesota, 2000–2018. Med Care 2021;59:S220. https://doi.org/10.1097/MLR.0000000000001435.

16. Henwood BF, Byrne T, Scriber B. Examining mortality among formerly homeless adults enrolled in Housing First: An observational study. BMC Publ Health 2015;15(1):1–8.

17. Becker JN, Foli KJ. Health-seeking behaviours in the homeless population: A concept analysis. Health Soc Care Community 2022;30(2):e278–86.

18. Schiltz NK, Chagin K, Sehgal AR. Clustering of Social Determinants of Health Among Patients - Nicholas K. Schiltz, Kevin Chagin, Ashwini R. Sehgal, 2022. Available at: https://journals.sagepub.com/doi/full/10.1177/21501319221113543. Accessed September 13, 2023.

19. Fernandez SB, Lopez C, Ibarra C, et al. Examining barriers to medication adherence and retention in care among women living with HIV in the face of homelessness and unstable housing. Int J Environ Res Publ Health 2022;19(18):11484.

20. Wadhera RK, Khatana SAM, Choi E, et al. Disparities in care and mortality among homeless adults hospitalized for cardiovascular conditions. JAMA Intern Med 2020;180(3):357–66.

21. Fan Q, Nogueira L, Yabroff KR, et al. Housing and cancer care and outcomes: a systematic review. JNCI: J Natl Cancer Inst 2022;114(12):1601–18.

22. Leifheit KM, Schwartz GL, Pollack CE, et al. Severe housing insecurity during pregnancy: association with adverse birth and infant outcomes. Int J Environ Res Publ Health 2020;17(22):8659.

23. Logie CH, Sokolovic N, Kazemi M, et al. Does resource insecurity drive HIV-related stigma? Associations between food and housing insecurity with HIV-related stigma in cohort of women living with HIV in Canada. J Int AIDS Soc 2022;25:e25913.

24. Benfer EA, Vlahov D, Long MY, et al. Eviction, health inequity, and the spread of COVID-19: housing policy as a primary pandemic mitigation strategy. J Urban Health 2021;98:1–12.

25. Felt D, Xu J, Floresca YB, et al. Instability in housing and medical care access: the inequitable impacts of the COVID-19 pandemic on US transgender populations. Transgender Health 2023;8(1):74–83.

26. Green H, Fernandez R, MacPhail C. The social determinants of health and health outcomes among adults during the COVID-19 pandemic: a systematic review. Publ Health Nurs 2021;38(6):942–52.

27. McLeroy KR, Bibeau D, Steckler A, et al. An ecological perspective on health promotion programs. Health Educ Q 1988;15(4):351–77. https://doi.org/10.1177/109019818801500401.

28. Valdez A. Words matter: Labelling, bias and stigma in nursing. J Adv Nurs 2021;77(11):e33–5.

29. Hamann HA, Ostroff JS, Marks EG, et al. Stigma among patients with lung cancer: A patient-reported measurement model. Psycho Oncol 2014;23(1):81–92.

30. Nyblade L, Stangl A, Weiss E, et al. Combating HIV stigma in health care settings: what works? J Int AIDS Soc 2009;12:1–7.
31. Ross CA, Goldner EM. Stigma, negative attitudes and discrimination towards mental illness within the nursing profession: a review of the literature. J Psychiatr Ment Health Nurs 2009;16(6):558–67.
32. Bronfenbrenner U. Toward an experimental ecology of human development. Am Psychol 1977;32(7):513–31. https://doi.org/10.1037/0003-066X.32.7.513.
33. Biederman DJ, Nichols TR. Homeless women's experiences of service provider encounters. J Community Health Nurs 2014;31(1):34–48.
34. Gunner E, Chandan SK, Marwick S, et al. Provision and accessibility of primary healthcare services for people who are homeless: a qualitative study of patient perspectives in the UK. Br J Gen Pract 2019;69(685):e526–36. https://doi.org/10.3399/bjgp19X704633.
35. Goddu AP, O'Conor KJ, Lanzkron S, et al. Do words matter? Stigmatizing language and the transmission of bias in the medical record. J Gen Intern Med 2018;33:685–91.
36. Barker SL, Maguire N. Experts by experience: peer support and its use with the homeless. Community Ment Health J 2017;53:598–612.
37. Tan Z, Mun EY, Nguyen USD, et al. Increases in social support co-occur with decreases in depressive symptoms and substance use problems among adults in permanent supportive housing: an 18-month longitudinal study. BMC psychology 2021;9:1–13.
38. Joint Commission. New Requirements to Reduce Health Care Disparities. Published online June 20, 2022.
39. Fraze TK, Brewster AL, Lewis VA, et al. Prevalence of screening for food insecurity, housing instability, utility needs, transportation needs, and interpersonal violence by US physician practices and hospitals. JAMA Netw Open 2019;2(9):e1911514.
40. Montgomery A.E., Using a Universal Screener to Identify Veterans Experiencing Housing Instability. Published online March 2014. Available at: https://www.va.gov/HOMELESS/Universal_Screener_to_Identify_Veterans_Experiencing_Housing_Instability_2014.pdf.
41. American Hospital Association. ICD-10-CM Coding for Social Determinants of Health. Published January 2022. Available at: https://www.cms.gov/files/document/zcodes-infographic.pdf. Accessed September 14, 2023.
42. Centers for Medicare and Medicaid Services. ICD-10-CM Official Guidelines for Coding and Reporting. Published April 1, 2022. Available at: https://www.cms.gov/files/document/fy-2022-icd-10-cm-coding-guidelines-updated-02012022.pdf. Accessed September 14, 2023.
43. Best JA, Young A. A safe DC: a conceptual framework for care of the homeless inpatient. J Hosp Med 2009;4(6):375–81.
44. Greysen SR, Allen R, Rosenthal MS, et al. Improving the quality of discharge care for the homeless: a patient-centered approach. J Health Care Poor Underserved 2013;24(2):444–55.
45. National Institute for Medical Respite Care. What Is Medical Respite Care? National Institute for Medical Respite Care. Published n.d. Available at: https://nimrc.org/medical-respite/. Accessed September 14, 2023.
46. National Institute for Medical Respite Care. Medical Respite Care Directory. National Institute for Medical Respite Care. Published n.d. Available at: https://nimrc.org/medical-respite-directory/. Accessed September 14, 2023.
47. Biederman DJ, Gamble J, Wilson S, et al. Health care utilization following a homeless medical respite pilot program. Public Health Nurs 2019;36(3):296–302. https://doi.org/10.1111/phn.12589.

48. Biederman DJ, Sloane R, Gamble J, et al. Program outcomes and health care utilization of people experiencing homelessness and substance use disorder after transitional care program engagement. J Health Care Poor Underserved 2021; 33(3):1337–52.
49. Hudson BF, Flemming K, Shulman C, et al. Challenges to access and provision of palliative care for people who are homeless: a systematic review of qualitative research. BMC Palliat Care 2016;15(1):1–18.
50. National Homeless Law Center. Housing not Handcuffs, 2021: State Law Supplement. Published November 2021. Available at: https://homelesslaw.org/wp-content/uploads/2021/11/2021-HNH-State-Crim-Supplement.pdf. Accessed September 14, 2023.
51. Housing PLUS Act of 2023 (H.R. 3405). Available at: https://www.govtrack.us/congress/bills/118/hr3405. Accessed September 15, 2023.

Facilitating Gender-Affirming Nursing Encounters

Ethan C. Cicero, PhD, RN[a],*, Jordon D. Bosse, PhD, RN[b],
Dallas Ducar, MSN, RN, APRN, PMHNP-BC, CNL[c],
Christine Rodriguez, DNP, APRN, FNP-BC, MDiv, MA[d],
Jess Dillard-Wright, PhD, MA, RN, CNM[e]

KEYWORDS

- Nursing • Gender-affirming care • Transgender • Gender identity
- Nursing assessment

KEY POINTS

- Gender-affirming care (GAC) is delivered through interpersonal interactions and with the provision of multifaceted interventions that affirm and validate an individual's gender identity and gender expression.
- Gender affirmation, including the delivery of GAC, is a social determinant of health for transgender, nonbinary, and other gender expansive (TNGE) people.
- Nurses possess the ability to provide GAC in any health care setting, for any type of health care encounter, and to all clients, including TNGE people.

INTRODUCTION

Everyone has a gender identity, that is, a sense of self and their gender: being a man, woman, both, neither, or something else entirely.[1] Gender identity is shaped by social, cultural, and political environments in which people are embedded, and it evolves across the lifespan.[1] As a social process, gender is structured according to narrowly defined gender norms that configure gender in a binary with "man" at one pole and "woman" at the other. However, gender is a developmental process that links the biological, psychological, and social in reciprocally reinforcing fashion that exists on a

[a] Emory University, Nell Hodgson Woodruff School of Nursing, 1520 Clifton Road, Atlanta, GA 30322, USA; [b] College of Nursing, University of Rhode Island, 350 Eddy Street, Providence, RI 02903, USA; [c] Transhealth, PO Box 9120, Chelsea, MA 02150, USA; [d] Yale School of Nursing, Yale University; 400 West Campus Drive, Orange, CT 06477, USA; [e] Elaine Marieb College of Nursing, University of Massachusetts Amherst, 130 Skinner Hall, 651 North Pleasant Street, Amherst, MA 01103, USA
* Corresponding author.
E-mail address: ethan.cicero@emory.edu

Nurs Clin N Am 59 (2024) 75–96
https://doi.org/10.1016/j.cnur.2023.11.007
0029-6465/24/© 2023 Elsevier Inc. All rights reserved.
nursing.theclinics.com

spectrum.[2] Gender affirmation occurs when a person's gender identity or gender expression is socially accepted and supported.[3] Within health care settings and by health care professionals, this confirmation process is described as gender-affirming care (GAC).[4] Most often, GAC is associated with transgender, nonbinary, and other gender expansive (TNGE) people. However, the health care that cisgender people receive consistently affirms cisnormative gender expectations. Consider the soft lighting and pink gowns offered by breast health centers, evoking femininity in the context of health care services or prescriptions to assure masculine virility like sildenafil for erectile dysfunction and finasteride for hair loss. This suggests that GAC is already a reality that exists and something that nurses do every day for their cisgender clients. Nurses possess the ability to provide GAC to all clients, but they may feel unprepared and uninformed in how to translate their knowledge and skills into the provision of GAC for TNGE people.[5]

The purpose of this article is to highlight the essentials for facilitating gender-affirming nursing encounters for TNGE folks. As such, this article will not be exhaustive—a single paper cannot and will not provide all knowledge, insight, and guidance to account for the vast and disparate health care needs of all TNGE people across all areas of nursing in every type of health care environment. Second, although gender and sexuality are related, they are also distinct, and we are focused on gender identities. To accomplish our purpose, we first lay out some shared language to work from which gives way to a brief overview of the stigma and discrimination that structure TNGE people's lives and health care experiences, which has a considerable impact on their health. This is particularly relevant in a time of increasing state scrutiny, policing, violence, and discrimination directed toward TNGE people. We then illustrate what constitutes as gender-affirming nursing encounters by characterizing gender-affirming approaches to conducting and documenting a nursing assessment and describing techniques to overcome institutional-level challenges that may hinder a nurse's ability in establishing gender-affirming therapeutic relationships with TNGE people. Finally, we provide strategies that nurses can use to improve their health care organization and interprofessional collaborative practice to create psychologically and physically safe health care spaces for TNGE people. We begin by defining our terms.

Defining Our Terms

As we articulate our vision for gender-affirming nursing encounters, the discussion benefits from some definitions. The first concerns who we mean when we say "we." At first glance, this might seem like a straightforward or unnecessary explanation. However, when we use the word "we," each of us as authors is connected to different communities, different realities, and different experiences. This introduces ambiguity that can be confusing. For the purposes of this article, when we use "we," we are referring to ourselves as an authorial collective. For other communities, including ones of which we are a part, we name them specifically: nurses, advanced practice nurses, Indigenous and People of Color, queer folks, transgender people, genderqueer humans, disabled folks, scholars, parents, partners, and so on.

We use the phrase "transgender, nonbinary, and gender expansive" (TNGE) to collectively describe people whose gender identity or expression differs from the sex assigned to them at birth. The TNGE population is sizable and growing, composed of considerable diversity and thus should not be understood as monolithic.[1,6] It includes individuals who self-identify within the gender binary like transgender women/men and transmasculine/transfeminine people as well as those who exist along or outside of the gender binary like agender, nonbinary, genderfluid, and genderqueer folks. There is considerable variation in terminology used to characterize and self-describe TNGE people.[1] Some may not use the term "transgender" to describe themselves and simply use man or woman. Terminology used to describe gender evolves with generational, geographic, and cultural variations.[1] For example, people who came to understand themselves as TNGE before the early 2000s may self-identify using terms like "transsexual," "female-to-male/FTM," or "male-to-female/MTF," terms that today are considered inappropriate by many.[7] Today, to achieve nuance and communicate additional information about who they are, individuals may use multiple terms to describe themselves.[8] Other relevant terms are defined in **Table 1**.

BACKGROUND

Although the term "transgender" is relatively new, TNGE *people* are not.[10] Gender as a category of identity is neither static nor stable across space and time given its socially constructed meaning and norms.[2] The gender binary is a product of colonialism and white supremacy.[11–13] Around the world and across time, gender has existed beyond binaries. Many cultures recognize a third gender. This includes Two-Spirit, a term used by some North American Indigenous communities to describe gender variant,[14] as well as *hijra* and *kothi,* South Asian descriptors for what folks in the United States would describe as transfeminine, nonbinary, and other gender expansive identities.[15] The impact of colonialism and the gender norms it produced gives increase to the notion that cisgender identities are normal, neutral, and natural, which leads to environments characterized by racism, phobia, and marginalization.[16] Health care is frequently one of the many spaces in which cisgender norms are disciplined and enforced, beginning with the assignment of sex at birth, a practice that is predominantly based on the appearance of external genitalia. This reproduces naturalized ideas about binary gender and the pathologization of TNGE identities.[13]

Gender Identity and Gender Incongruence

Gender identity is fluid, evolving over the lifespan.[1] Gender identity milestones, which may include feeling different about gender than expectations associated with sex assigned at birth, identifying as TNGE, living in their affirmed gender, and accessing gender-affirming medical interventions, occur at varying time points across the life course; gender identity is not a linear process.[17] Gender incongruence may first be experienced in childhood, late adulthood, or any time in between. It may be accompanied with significant distress known as gender dysphoria, which can be alleviated with a wide range of gender-affirming interventions.[1] Interventions include social approaches such as changes in names, pronouns, and gender expression, as well as medical interventions to delay puberty or achieve desired feminization/masculinization, surgeries to alter secondary sex characteristics and/or genitalia, and psychotherapy to promote resilience. Evidence-based approaches to address gender incongruence, outlined within the World Professional Association for Transgender Health's Standards of Care for the Health of Transgender and Gender Diverse People,[1] are described in **Table 2**.

Stigma and Discrimination

TGNE people experience stigma at structural, interpersonal, and individual levels, which can result in being treated with prejudice or experiencing discrimination.[21] Structural stigma refers to the societal norms and institutional policies, including those within health care organizations that reinforce gender binaries.[21] This form of stigma

Table 1
Terminology associated with transgender, nonbinary, and other gender expansive people

Cisgender	An adjective that describes people with an alignment between their sex assigned at birth aligns and gender identity.
Gender affirmation	An interpersonal, interactive process where an individual's gender identity or gender expression is socially accepted and supported.
Gender dysphoria	A diagnostic condition included in the Diagnostic and Statistical Manual of Mental Disorders (DSM), Fifth Edition, to describe clinically significant distress or impairment in social, occupation, or other areas of functioning due to a marked incongruence between one's experienced/expressed gender and primary and/or secondary sex characteristics (or in young adolescents, the anticipated secondary sex characteristics). The DSM includes a specific and separate set of criteria for children, adolescents, and adults.
Gender euphoria	A subjective experience, the "joyful feeling of rightness in one's gender"[9(p286)] and can result from interventions as simple as feeling "right" in clothes to consistently being referred by correct name and pronouns.
Gender expansive	"An adjective often used to describe people who identify or express themselves in ways that broaden the socially and culturally defined behaviors or beliefs associated with a particular sex."[1(pS252)]
Gender expression	Outward expression of gender through a combination of behaviors and mannerisms that includes name, pronouns, clothing, haircut, voice, body language, and other physical attributes.
Gender identity	A sense of self and their gender: being a man, woman, both, neither, or something else entirely, and it evolves across the lifespan
Gender incongruence	"A diagnostic term used in the International Classification of Diseases-11 that describes a person's marked and persistent experience of an incompatibility between that person's gender identity and the gender expected of them based on their birth-assigned sex." [1(pS252)]
Nonbinary	An adjective that "refers to those with gender identities outside the gender binary. People with nonbinary gender identities may identify as partially a man and partially a woman or identify as sometimes a man and sometimes a woman, or identify as a gender other than a man or a woman, or as not having a gender at all. Nonbinary people may use the pronouns they/them/theirs instead of he/him/his or she/her/hers. Some nonbinary people consider themselves to be transgender; some do not because they consider transgender to be part of the gender binary. Examples of nonbinary gender identities may include genderqueer, gender diverse, genderfluid, demigender, bigender, and agender."[1(pS252)]
Sex assigned at birth	Sex is determined and assigned at birth based primarily on the appearance of external genitalia. AFAB is an abbreviation for "assigned female at birth." AMAB is an abbreviation for "assigned male at birth."
Transfeminine	An adjective to describe individuals who identify on the feminine gender spectrum and were assigned male at birth.[4]
Transgender	An adjective that describes individuals with a gender identity that does not align with the sex they were assigned at birth.
Transition	"A process whereby people usually change from the gender expression associated with their assigned sex at birth to another gender expression that better matches their gender identity. People may transition socially by using methods such as changing their name,

(continued on next page)

Table 1 (continued)	
	pronoun, clothing, hair styles, and/or the ways that they move and speak. Transitioning may or may not involve hormones and/or surgeries to alter the physical body. Transition can be used to describe the process of changing one's gender expression from any gender to a different gender. People may transition more than once in their lifetimes."[1(pS253)]
	Transition is not a linear process from one gender to another gender; the only ideal "endpoint" is what the TNGE person identifies as necessary to feel at home in their body.
Transmasculine	An adjective to describe individuals who identify on the masculine gender spectrum and were assigned female at birth.[4]
Two-Spirit	An umbrella term, used by Native and Indigenous communities in the United States and Canada, to describe Indigenous peoples who are diverse in terms of their sexual orientation and gender identity

devalues, erases, or pathologizes TNGE people, sanctioning violence against TNGE communities through policies and legislation. Institutionally supported interventions to promote cisgenderism, or to "cure" gender nonconformity, is an example of structural stigma.[13] Structural stigma leads to the denial of health insurance coverage or benefits for necessary and preventative health care; limited or deficient training and curricula content provided to health care professionals; and legislation designed to strip TNGE people of protections against discrimination and basic human rights. Diagnostic labeling of TNGE identities as disorders is another example of structural stigma.[22] Although being transgender is no longer considered a mental health condition,[23] it was classified as a mental health condition until 2013 in the Diagnostic and Statistical Manual of Mental Disorders and as a mental disorder in the International Classification of Diseases until 2019.[22]

Interpersonal stigma is direct or enacted forms of stigma, which includes verbal harassment, physical violence, and sexual assault.[21] TNGE people experience higher rates of violence and discrimination while in school, on the job, and at the hands of their immediate family members and romantic partners.[20] Interpersonal stigma can also include other seemingly less harmful "mistakes" such as calling someone by the wrong name or pronouns as well as intentionally misgendering or ridiculing a person's gender expression. Because interpersonal stigma is reinforced by structural stigma, TNGE people, particularly transgender women of color are at high risk of fatal violence. Nearly 90% of TNGE victims of violence are transgender women and Black transgender women account for the majority of all known victims of fatal anti-transgender violence since 2013.[24] TNGE individuals are exposed to interpersonal stigma in all areas of life and many experience discrimination, mistreatment, or violence in public settings.[20]

At the individual level, stigma can affect TNGE individuals' psychological processes.[21] TNGE people may internalize negative thoughts and feelings about themselves called internalized transphobia, which may lead TNGE individuals to hide their gender identity or gender history. In addition, TNGE individuals may anticipate and expect rejection or discrimination from others, leading to decreased self-efficacy and ability to cope with stigma-related stressors.[25] As a self-protection strategy, TNGE people may become hypervigilant about encountering discrimination and avoid social interactions, including health care encounters.[25] They have good reason to anticipate this injustice: Within health care environments, TNGE encounter

Table 2

Gender affirmation: A multidimensional social determinant of transgender, nonbinary, and other gender expansive health. *Notes:* Gender affirmation is a social process where individuals, their gender identity, and gender expression are accepted, supported, and affirmed. It is also a multidimensional social determinant of health that improves physical and mental health outcomes, well-being, and overall quality of life for TNGE people.[1,4] Gender affirmation is person-centered, and no single approach or predetermined set of interventions defines what it is to be TNGE.[1,4] Within health care environments, GAC is delivered through interpersonal interactions and in partnership with the TNGE person to holistically support them in achieving desired health and well-being outcomes with the provision of multifaceted interventions that affirm and validate an individual's gender identity and gender expression.[1] It is vital that nurses understand that there is no one-size-fits-all approach to care for all TNGE people. Although some may choose gender-affirming medical interventions, others may feel relief simply with a social gender affirmation process. It may be helpful to conceptualize gender affirmation within four dimensions: social, psychological, legal, and medical gender affirmation.[4] We provide a description of and nursing implications for each dimension of gender affirmation.

Dimension	Description	Nursing Implications
Social gender affirmation	Nonmedical interventions that align an individual's gender within society. These approaches *may* include, but are not limited to changes to one's name, pronouns, and gender expression. Individuals may also use diet, exercise, and gender-affirming garments (ie, packers, gaffes, binders, and hip and buttocks pads) to shape their bodies, address dysphoria, and promote gender euphoria. Chest binding can create a flatter appearance to the chest by compressing the breast tissue. This can be accomplished using a commercial binder, sport bras, layering of shirts or sport bras, elastic bandages, athletic or kinesiology tape, or a combination of the above. Genital tucking is the practice of positioning the penis and testes to reduce the outward appearance of a genital bulge. This can be accomplished with underwear or a gaff. Other garments like packers and padding can be placed inside of clothing to create the appearance of a genital bulge or enhance the appearance of breasts, hips, or buttocks.	• Ensure chosen name and pronouns are used during all client encounters and when referring to the client with their extended treatment team. • Examine skin for breakdown related to chest binding or genital tucking. • Educate clients on safe chest binding practices to ensure adequate tidal volume can be achieved, breathing and blood flow are not restricted, and risk of skin breakdown and infection are minimized. • Educate clients on safe tucking practices to minimize the risk of skin breakdown and infection. • Encourage clients to allow time each day where they do not wear constricting garments and discourage them from wearing constricting garments while sleeping. • Assess for disordered eating behaviors and unhealthy exercise routines. Educate clients on healthy diet and exercise practices. • Social gender affirmation improves health outcomes.

Psychological gender affirmation	The goal of psychological gender affirmation is to promote resilience. This type of gender affirmation places emphasis on the individual's lived experiences on how they perceive and value oneself as a TNGE person, the comfort within their own bodies, as well as with their gender identity and gender expression. A range of psychotherapeutic frameworks can promote resilience, reduce internalized stigma, and assist the TNGE person in being respected and validated.	• Maintain a list of TGNE-friendly behavioral health resources, including providers, support groups, and TNGE community-serving organizations. • Remember that TNGE individuals do not *need* therapy because of their gender; rather therapy can support the TNGE person adjust to changes and provide support in dealing with the responses to external circumstances and adverse societal conditions. • Therapy that attempts to reverse or correct one's TNGE identity and make them more comfortable with their assigned sex at birth (ie, conversion therapy) is harmful and should never be recommended.
Legal gender affirmation	This type of affirmation includes updating legal documents with the individual's chosen name and correct gender marker. This *may* include changes to driver's licenses, social security cards, birth certificates, and passports. Legal gender affirmation can help TNGE people move through the world more safely by improving access to employment, housing, education, health care, and social services.[18] Not only do these legal changes serve to affirm and validate TNGE individuals, but they also serve as a psychological safety measure. For example, having affirming legal documentation may help someone feel more confident in themselves and their identity.[19]	• Provide local resources to support legal gender affirmation (**Table 3**). • Update EHR to reflect legal changes to name and gender marker. • Nurses should be aware of the laws and policies for the state where they practice for changing names and gender markers on legal documents. Whether someone can change their gender marker on their birth certificate or other legal documents, and the requirements to do so, vary by state. Several states have a nonbinary "X" gender marker option (see **Table 3**).
Medical gender affirmation	Medical gender affirmation includes medical and surgical interventions to ameliorate gender dysphoria experienced by TNGE people and support gender euphoria. Medical interventions *may* include: • Pubertal suppression with gonadotropin-releasing hormone agonists • Masculinizing hormones with testosterone • Feminizing hormones with estrogen formulations, progestogens, and antiandrogens	• Nurses should be knowledgeable about gender-affirming hormone therapy and gender-affirming surgeries, which is outlined below. Additionally, nurses should become familiar with their local clinics and providers who can provide gender-affirming medical and surgical interventions in the event that a patient requests a referral for such care. • Pubertal suppression is reversible. If someone stops taking blockers, puberty associated with their sex assigned at birth will resume.

(continued on next page)

Table 2
(continued)

- Facial hair removal
- Vocal therapy
- Surgical interventions *may* include:
- Chest contouring or mastectomy (with or without nipple graft), or mammoplasty (ie, "top" surgery)
- Hysterectomy/oophorectomy or orchiectomy
- Genital surgery such as vaginoplasty, vulvoplasty; metoidioplasty, or phalloplasty, with or without scrotoplasty (ie, "bottom" surgery)
- Facial feminization surgery
- Vocal cord surgery
- Hair restoration/transplantation

- The use of gender-affirming hormone therapy is a lifelong commitment for most TNGE people. Clients receiving these exogenous sex hormones will require continuous laboratory monitoring (eg, total testosterone, estradiol levels, CBC).
- Laboratory reference ranges for the individual's affirmed gender should be used for clients on gender-affirming hormone therapy.[1]
- There are various routes, formulations, and dosing for gender-affirming hormone therapy (eg, subcutaneous, intramuscular, transdermal, oral, sublingual).
- Educate TNGE clients on the appropriate and safe administration of hormonal treatments.
- Although not everyone desires medical or surgical interventions, many who do may not have access to such interventions due to financial reasons or other structural barriers such as provider gatekeeping and anti-TNGE legislation.[20]
- Surgical interventions, particularly genital surgery, among adolescents are very rare. Social transitions are recommended for prepubescent youth.[1]
- Very few TNGE people regret their medical/surgical gender affirmation.[1]

Abbreviations: ACE, adverse childhood experience; CBC, complete blood count; EHR, electronic health record; GAC, gender-affirming care; TNGE, transgender, nonbinary, and gender expansive.

Table 3
Resources

Organization	Description
Center for Urban Pedagogy	Show Up, a useful resource for how to intervene when someone else is being harassed. https://www.sfzc.org/files/ShowUp-BystanderIntervention
GLMA: Health Professionals Advancing LGBTQ + Equality*	Professional association of LGBTQ+ and allied health professionals, which includes a nursing section. They focus on research, advocacy, and education. GLMA offers webinars, conferences, online educational modules, an LGBTQ + friendly provider list, and resources for LGBTQ + clients. www.glma.org
Human Rights Campaign Healthcare Equality Index	Guidance on policies and practices which are inclusive of LGBTQ + clients, visitors, and employees, with specific resources available for Veteran's and Children's hospitals. https://www.thehrcfoundation.org/professional-resources/hei-resource-guide Institutions can also apply for recognition for their inclusive policies through the Healthcare Equality Index https://www.thehrcfoundation.org/professional-resources/hei-scoring-criteria
Lambda Legal	Creating Equal Access to Quality Health Care for Transgender Patients: Transgender-Affirming Hospital Policies https://legacy.lambdalegal.org/publications/fs_transgender-affirming-hospital-policies
Movement Advancement Project*	An independent, nonprofit think tank focused on creating an inclusive and equitable America. They provide equality maps that track over 50 different LGBTQ-related laws and policies, including those associated with name changes and gender marker updates on driver's license, birth certificates, and other legal documents. https://www.lgbtmap.org/
National Center for Transgender Equality*	Provides guidance on policy and legal issues for TNGE folks, including state-level name change processes. https://transequality.org/documents
National League for Nursing: Advancing Care Excellence for the LGBTQ + People (ACE+)	The ACE project provides evidence-based teaching resources about nursing care for LGBTQ + people. The overarching goal of this project is to equip nurse educators with the necessary tools to teach care of LGBTQ + people and help them graduate a new nursing workforce that is both knowledgeable and culturally informed to meet the needs of LGBTQ + individuals and decrease the health disparities they experience. https://www.nln.org/education/teaching-resources/professional-development-programsteaching-resourcesace-all/aceplus
National LGBT Cancer Network*	Provides culturally relevant information for cancer screening, tobacco cessation, training materials, resources to identify inclusive screening providers and treatment services and caregiver resources. https://cancer-network.org/

(continued on next page)

Table 3 (continued)	
Organization	**Description**
National LGBT Health Education Center at The Fenway Institute	National LGBT Health Education Center hosts annual "Advancing Excellence in Transgender Health" Conference; resources for clients and providers https://fenwayhealth.org/the-fenway-institute/education/the-national-lgbtia-health-education-center/
SAGE	Advocacy and services for LGBTQ + elders. www.sageusa.org
Sexual Orientation and Gender Identity Nursing	Created by an interdisciplinary group of professionals and academics from Canada, the Web site is a toolkit for nurses and nursing educators committed to providing resources and education in health care. https://soginursing.ca
Trans Lifeline*	24/7, phone-based crisis support for TNGE adults (English and Spanish). They also provide resources for community-based peer support, navigating legal processes such as name changes and microgrants to help TNGE people access legal services and gender-affirming interventions. https://translifeline.org/hotline/
Transline	Provides consultation for medical professionals. http://project-health.org/transline
Transgender Training Institute	Guide to pronouns. https://www.transgendertraininginstitute.com/resources/pronouns/
The Trevor Project*	Provides 24/7 phone and text-based crisis support for LGBTQ + young people. https://www.thetrevorproject.org/
UCSF Gender Affirming Health Program	Publishes the "Guidelines for the primary and gender-affirming care of transgender and gender nonbinary people" https://transcare.ucsf.edu/guidelines and hosts the biannual conference, "National Transgender Health Summit" https://prevention.ucsf.edu/transhealth
World Professional Association for Transgender Health	An international, multidisciplinary, professional association that promotes evidence-based care, education, research, public policy, and respect in transgender health. www.wpath.org

Abbreviation: LGBTQ+, lesbian, gay, bisexual, transgender, queer/questioning, and other non-heterosexual and/or non-cisgender identities.

discrimination, harassment, physical violence, and care refusal from clinicians, nurses, and other health care professionals,[20,26] with nonbinary individuals and those with a nonconforming gender expression facing more discrimination than binary identifying/appearing people.[27] As a form of self-preservation, some TNGE individuals with a gender expression concordant with social norms and who are assumed to cisgender may choose to avoid disclosing their TNGE identity to health care providers, and as a result, they may not receive preventative care associated with anatomy they may still possess like prostate examinations for transgender women and Pap tests for transgender men.[25]

Social and Health Inequities

Stigma assigned to TNGE folks gives increase to social and health inequities.[28] All too often, scholarship focused on TNGE health wallows in trauma, replicating deficit models of health outcomes inequity. Here, we wish to squarely focus our gaze on the institutions, structures, and systems that produce and reinforce these inequities. Health care pathologizes TNGE people and is implicated in the larger social project that produces stigma and discriminatory encounters as outlined above.[29] Stigma exacerbates social inequities experienced by TNGE folks. TNGE people are more likely to experience poverty because of stigma assigned to their gender identity, despite achieving higher levels of education than their cisgender counterparts.[30] In turn, TNGE people being more likely to be uninsured[31] and experience housing instability or be unhoused.[20,32] These inequities are compounded by other forms of oppression such as racism, ageism, sexism, homophobia, classism, and ableism. Within the TNGE population, those from minoritized ethnoracial groups experience higher rates of homelessness, unemployment, and lack of health insurance when compared with their white TNGE counterparts.[20]

Stigma is a significant source of stress that drives health inequities for TNGE people. Although health inequities, such as social inequalities, experienced by TNGE people vary considerably by TNGE community,[33] the TNGE population experience higher levels of anxiety and depression, worse physical health, and are more likely to have multiple chronic health conditions, again a function of systemic and structural oppression.[34,35] Chronic exposure to stigma and discrimination can cause or exacerbate socially induced health problems and chronic health conditions as well as contribute toward unhealthy aging.[1,36]

GENDER-AFFIRMING NURSING ENCOUNTERS

Gender affirmation, including the provision of GAC, is a social determinant of TNGE health.[4] TNGE individuals should be affirmed in all aspects of life. Nurses can deliver GAC in any health care setting and for any type of health care encounter. The delivery of GAC may not always be straightforward and prescriptive. This is precisely where its strength lies. GAC is holistic, comprehensive, and person-centered, congruent with the emancipatory and social justice aims of nursing care.[37] GAC allows care recipients, or clients, and their nurses to explore gender euphoria,[9] promoting wellness in a way that health care often neglects. Gender euphoria is a subjective experience, the "joyful feeling of rightness in one's gender"[9(p286)] and can result from interventions as simple as feeling "right" in clothes to consistently being referred by correct name and pronouns. Too often, health care engenders gender dysphoria by pathologizing bodies and identities, pushing individuals into predefined boxes shaped by white cisheteropatriarchy and imperialism. GAC challenges this paradigm, ceding power, and control of health care to the client. This enables TNGE people to make informed decisions about their bodies, identities, and ultimately their health and well-being. By virtue of the intimacy of nursing care, nurses are uniquely positioned to induce gender euphoria by delivering GAC. Nurses can partner with their clients in shaping the health care experience where the client is the expert about their gender and the nurse provides expertise in nursing care.

Psychosocial Considerations for Establishing a Gender-Affirming Therapeutic Relationship

Before outlining gender-affirming approaches to conducting a nursing assessment, we first provide some broad psychosocial considerations in establishing a therapeutic nursing relationship with the client. It may take longer to build a therapeutic connection and trust with TNGE clients because it is likely they have been mistreated in health care.[26] Although a helpful approach with all clients, it may be particularly important to use trauma-informed approaches when working with TNGE people because of the extent of discrimination-related trauma experienced by the population. Delivering care with a trauma-informed approach means recognizing the widespread impacts of trauma and its potential symptoms and working to prevent re-traumatization. Creating a care environment that is emotionally safe is critical to the nursing assessment and the top priority of trauma-informed care.

Beginning the Care Encounter

To set the stage for a GAC encounter, nurses should start all care encounters by introducing themselves by providing their name and pronouns and then inviting the client to do the same. This gesture creates intimacy and fosters a sense of safety in addressing gender-related care considerations. Ensuing care encounters and during all interactions, nurses should always use the client-provided name and pronouns. Some people may not use pronouns, or some may choose not to share their pronouns; in this case, ask the client how they would like to be addressed, "what would you like me to call you?" This approach invites clients to share while avoiding misnaming or misgendering them. A nurse engaging with TNGE clients may make mistakes and use the wrong name or pronoun. The key is to apologize once for the mistake, correct the error, and use the correct language in subsequent interactions.[38]

Some nurses may feel uncomfortable asking about gender identity, think it is irrelevant,[39] or worry that they will offend their clients.[39,40] Most people do not feel offended when asked about their identities, understand the importance of providing the information, and are comfortable disclosing their identities.[41,42] Knowing clients' identities allows nurses to both improve their relationships with them and to ensure the highest quality care is provided.[43]

If the client is accompanied by someone, the nurse should ask about their relationship rather than making assumptions. Nurses may care for TNGE persons with unsupportive caregivers, partners, or children who are referring to the client by something other than the client's request while present in the treatment room. In this situation, it is important to give the TNGE person a choice about how they want the nurse to respond. Using the TNGE person's chosen name and pronouns with those who are not accepting is an opportunity for the nurse to model affirming behavior to unsupportive individuals. However, this approach could also cause more problems for the client by potentially adding strain in their relationship with the unsupportive person or even, a loss of financial support. The TNGE client may want the nurse to use their chosen name when they are alone, use a family nickname if family members or friends are present, or avoid using pronouns altogether. Until the nurse can confirm the client's choice, the nurse should use a gender neutral approach when speaking with caregivers or family members, referring to the client as "your child" versus "son/daughter," "partner" versus "husband/wife," or "they" versus "he/she."

Gender-Affirming Nursing Assessments

The nursing assessment is a systematic collection of information about an individual's health status that includes information about health history and physical assessment. When performing a nursing assessment, nurses should ensure the client understands why the questions are being asked, who will have access to their responses, and why it might be necessary to share the information. As the nurse completes a health history and physical examination, their assessment should focus on what is immediately relevant care. It is never acceptable to ask questions out of curiosity about a TNGE person's birth name, gender-affirming hormone therapy, surgical history, or pursuit of other gender-affirming interventions. If history-taking involves necessary questions about topics that are often stigmatized or may provoke feelings of shame or guilt, such as sexual health history or substance use patterns, explain to the client that the questions are asked of everyone. This strategy normalizes stigmatized topics and distances them from TNGE identity; this may make the client more comfortable answering the questions.[44] If a client is accompanied by anyone, be sure to ask if they are comfortable answering sensitive questions with the visitor present; if necessary, direct the visitor to a waiting area to facilitate privacy.

Throughout the assessment, if the client uses unfamiliar language to describe some aspect of their identity, anatomy, or health-related behavior, ask the client to clarify what the term(s) means to them. The use of gender neutral language and open-ended questions throughout the assessment allow the nurse to take a more inclusive approach in collecting pertinent information. For example, asking, "who are the important people in your life?" provides information about the client's support network. At the end of the history-taking, the nurse should summarize key points, providing the client with an opportunity to correct or clarify anything the nurse may have misunderstood and provide any additional information. These additional steps help ensure the nurse obtained accurate, relevant information before moving on to the physical assessment.

Gender-Affirming Physical Assessments

The physical assessment portion of an examination may be a full head-to-toe assessment, or a more focused, system-specific assessment based on the reason for the visit. In either case, a systematic approach is helpful. Physical assessments may be especially challenging for some TNGE people due to prior negative health care experiences or gender dysphoria. The following are strategies to mitigate harm and affirm gender while conducting a trauma-informed physical assessment with TNGE folks.

- Ask the client if they would like to have a support person present and/or if they are comfortable with you doing the examination. They may prefer someone of a different gender.
- Give the client a choice when sensitive areas will be assessed. They may prefer to have this examination conducted first or at the end of the physical assessment.
- Use gender neutral language like groin instead of penis or vagina and chest instead of breasts when discussing genitals and sex-related characteristics. Some TNGE people use medical terms to refer to genitalia, but others either avoid using specific terminology or may use alternate language like "genitals" or "front hole" instead of "vagina."[45] When the nurse needs to talk about or examine genitalia, they can ask the client what, if any, specific language they would like the nurse to use. Mirror the language used by the client whenever possible.
- Clients should only be asked to take off as much clothing as necessary. This includes any gender-affirming garments such as chest binders, compression shirts, and shape-forming undergarments. If a gender-affirming garment must be temporarily removed for part of the assessment, the nurse should give the client privacy to do so and provide them time to put the garment(s) back on before continuing with the examination.

- Obtain client consent before touching their body, before beginning the physical assessment, and throughout the care encounter.
- Provide anticipatory guidance by informing the client what to expect throughout the assessment: "You're going to feel my hand [describe location], now you're going to feel an alcohol wipe, it might feel cold."
- Encourage clients to collect their own sample, when possible, especially for invasive assessments like Pap tests or frontal human papillomavirus specimen collection among transmasculine people. This may enhance comfort and make folks more likely to complete the test.[46,47]
- Stop health care rubbernecking. TNGE people are often put on "display" in health care settings by the professionals caring for them. TNGE people and their bodies are not "learning experiences" and should not be objectified as such.[48,49]
- Secure permission from a TNGE client *before* bringing in a nursing student or another individual in training and make sure the client understands that they have the right to refuse the request.

Documenting the Assessment

Electronic health record (EHR) systems are all different. Some institutions may not have a place to document someone's chosen name, pronouns, and/or gender identity. Others may have these fields available, but do not provide adequate response options. It also may be difficult to find where in the EHR this information is, or should be, documented. Nurses should familiarize themselves with their institution's EHR system to determine whether, and where, this information as well as an organ inventory can be documented. An organ inventory is a checklist of what organs a client does and does not have. This guides the provision of high-quality and appropriate preventive and maintenance health care.[50] Having an organ inventory can remind a clinician to conduct an annual prostate examination for transgender women who still have a prostate.[50] The use of an organ inventory can also prevent unnecessary examinations, laboratories, or procedures like a pregnancy test or Pap examination for a transmasculine person with a history of a total hysterectomy.[51] It is important to verify EHR data annually and update the record to reflect any changes in gender identity, name, pronouns, and anatomy because these items may evolve over the lifespan.[51]

Although it is important to ask everyone about their identities, including sexual orientation and gender identity, not everyone will want to share that information or have it documented in their chart.[52] When unsure whether a client has concerns about specific aspects of their identity or experience being documented, ask for clarification and confirm what will be documented. For example, if a TNGE adolescent or young adult who is still under their guardian's health insurance had concerns about their guardian finding out their identity, confidentiality can be maintained by using gender neutral language within nursing documentation. Similarly, there is no need to disclose a client's TNGE status or mention sex assigned at birth in narrative notes if it is not relevant to the encounter.[52] Be particularly mindful that their documentation could be viewed by other individuals who should not be privy to the information. Clients have a right to see their EHR and may read the narrative notes charted by nursing staff. The use of stigmatizing language, the wrong name or pronouns, or gendered language inconsistent with the language the client uses is detrimental to the therapeutic relationship and may impact trust and engagement in the health care system.[52]

Potential Institutional Barriers to Consider

EHR and other hospital-based records systems within a facility might not talk to one another. For example, the system used by the registration department to create client identification bands may display the client's birth name or legal name. Nurses may not be able to change this. Nurses can advocate for TNGE clients by asking the registration department to reissue the identification band using the correct name. If this is not possible, nurses should communicate the name discrepancy to the charge nurse, during handoff reports, other members of the treatment team, and any ancillary staff member who will be interacting with the client like unit clerks, phlebotomists, physical and occupational therapists, clergy, and others in the health care milieu as well as writing the correct client name on the whiteboard inside of their room.[53] Client identification bands are often used to confirm a client's identity before medication administration or procedures out of convenience. However, other identifying information such as date of birth or telephone number that can be confirmed with the EHR is also acceptable.[54] Nurses can convey empathy by acknowledging an understanding of these challenges and areas of frustration for TNGE clients. Directly communicating these potential barriers and explaining what the nurse will do to address them can help foster trust and establish a therapeutic relationship with TNGE clients.

Supporting Environmental and Institutional Inclusion of Diverse Gender Identities

Nurses can also work to create more welcoming health care environments in their specific unit and throughout their institution. We provide ways nurses can ensure their health care environments and colleagues are affirming to people of all gender identities in the following.

Create an affirming care environment: The health care environment can provide clues to how welcoming a space might be. It is not enough to create a safe environment by displaying visual symbols of inclusion, such as pride flags. Safe, welcoming, and inclusive environments that affirm the client's identity may include:

- Single-stall bathrooms designated as gender inclusive, noting anyone can use irrespective of their gender identity.
- Client-facing health promotion and education materials include images of information relevant to TNGE people.
- Intake forms and other documents used to collect health information include questions for clients to indicate their pronouns, sex assigned at birth, and self-identify their gender. Forms should include a range of inclusive gender identities and pronouns as well as a write-in option for both. Nurses should review the information before interacting with the client.[55]
- Nurses and all health care professionals can show they are a member of or an ally to the TNGE community by wearing a pin, sticker, lanyard, badge reel, or other accessories (eg, a rainbow, pink triangle, pronouns).
- Room TNGE individuals based on their gender identity, not their assigned sex at birth. For example, rather than placing a TNGE person scheduled for a hysterectomy on a gynecologic floor, they could be placed on a general medical-surgical floor. This protects their gender history and avoids discomfort for the TNGE client.
- When possible, room clients privately.[56]
- When sharing a room is necessary, discuss preferences, safety, and the possibility of delays with TNGE clients, particularly when hospital beds are limited.

Foster interprofessional collaboration: Nurses work collaboratively with all members of the health care team to coordinate GAC. This might involve participating in case conferences or team meetings, or referring clients to other professionals who specialize in TNGE health.

Serve as a resource. Become familiar with resources in your area specifically for TNGE people so you can provide relevant referrals or community resources. Given the increased risk of TNGE people experiencing discrimination and health care refusal, it could be helpful to assess providers' experience and willingness to care for TNGE people before providing referrals to them. This applies to general health care and TNGE-specific health care needs (see **Table 3** for resources).

GAC and continuous learning: Continuous learning is a key component of GAC. Nurses need to ensure they and their colleagues are educated on core concepts of GAC and how TNGE individuals thrive when they are provided appropriate and equitable health care. Other core education areas include the understanding of the common experience of clinicians relying on TNGE individuals to teach them about TNGE people, the health consequences stemming from receiving non-affirming care, experiencing discrimination and stigmatization, having insufficient or lacking adequate social support, and enduring the politicization of TNGE bodies and their human rights. Continuing education will create a stronger, more effective nurse advocate.

Be an advocate: Nurses are charged by the American Nurses Association Code of Ethics to act as advocates for their clients.[57] In a health care system that often marginalizes TNGE people, advocacy might involve standing up for a client's rights, ensuring their needs are met, and educating other members of the health care team about GAC. Nurses should correct other health care professionals if they use the wrong name or pronouns, make inappropriate statements when working with or talking about TNGE clients, or disclose someone's gender identity or gender history to others who do not need to know. Advocacy also means fighting for policy change at the institutional, local, state, and federal level. Advocate for the development of inclusive policies for TNGE clients and staff and encourage your organization to get recognition for policies and procedures that are inclusive and affirming to TNGE people, such as being listed on the Health Equality Index (see **Table 3**). Furthermore, if you are in a leadership position, recruit members of the TNGE community for roles in all areas of your health care organization.

DISCUSSION

In an effort to move from the "thoughts and prayers" of empty position statements decrying discrimination and violence against TNGE people that lack substantive, material interventions in the realities of health care,[58] with this article, we outline the essentials for facilitating gender-affirming nursing encounters. The actions outlined above constitute interventions nurses can make in their daily practice that represent a starting place for care that is affirming and safe. However, these practices are not the endpoint. In the discussion that follows, we outline critical next steps in the provision of GAC and building worlds in which TNGE folks can flourish.

GAC is life-saving care. This begins when the client first interacts with the health care facility, which might be the first time they physically enter the health care environment, calls the facility, accesses the hospital's Web site, or completes intake forms. By the time nurses enter the equation, clients may have already experienced transmisia—oppression, discrimination, or hatred of TNGE people[59]—in pursuit of health care. This means that although nursing-client interactions are so important, these interactions are not the only location in health care that requires transformation to ensure safe, atraumatic, and affirming care. Gender-affirming nursing care, like all nursing care, is situated and contextual,[60] with the nursing encounter at the most distal end of the downstream. This means that to create truly GAC environments, nurses must step outside the care encounter to examine, understand, and transform health care environments and organizations. This has implications for practice site policy at the most local level, evaluating and assessing the literature, Web presence, forms, TNGE community feedback, and processes of a given practice milieu to ensure that people have the best possible care experiences in that setting.

The implications for nursing do not stop with the practice environment, however. The provision of gender-affirming nursing care also comes with an ethical responsibility to speak up and actively resist local, state, and federal laws that infringe on the rights and well-being of all folks in nursing care.[57] Nurses are consistently rated the most trusted profession.[61] This political capital means that nurses are uniquely positioned to advocate for policies that foster health and well-being. In states where enacted laws target TNGE people, nurses must take a stand against unjust legislation precisely because it diminishes health and well-being. For individual nurses, this might look like safeguarding client records, providing necessary care regardless of legal threats, and being vocal opponents of policies that harm TNGE clients. It also means pushing professional nursing organizations to use their political capital to lobby for legislation that supports the health and well-being of transgender folks.[58]

Supporting GAC in health care environments demands authentic leadership that acknowledges, hears, affirms, and honors all voices.[62] This kind of leadership requires leaders to be true to themselves while fostering a climate where others feel comfortable expressing their true selves without fear of harm or retaliation. It also requires the kind of fearlessness that steps up, speaks truth to power, and does the right thing, even when it is daunting.[63] Practices of authentic leadership are linked to increased hope in health care settings,[64] a practice that is urgently needed for nursing in a time when burnout is rising and for TNGE folks in the face of eroding civil rights. Upholding nursing's commitment to dignity, well-being, and social justice demands a commitment to diversity, inclusion, justice, and equity. This extends beyond passive acceptance into active advocacy, necessitating an institutional culture that encourages learning, open dialogue, and respect for all identities.

SUMMARY

Gender-affirming nursing encounters are a social determinant of health for TNGE people. Nurses possess the ability to provide GAC in any health care setting, for any type of health care encounter, and to all clients, including TNGE people. GAC is holistic, comprehensive, and person-centered, congruent with the emancipatory and social justice aims of nursing care.

In a health care system that often marginalizes TNGE people, nurses can create a more welcoming and emotionally safe health care environment and act as advocates for TNGE clients. Advocacy involves standing up for a client's rights, ensuring their needs are met, educating other members of the health care team about GAC, and fighting for policy change at the institutional, local, state, and federal levels.

CLINICS CARE POINTS

- Trauma-informed approaches may be particularly important when working with transgender, nonbinary, and other gender expansive (TNGE) people due to high rates of health care discrimination-related trauma. Nurses must create physically and psychologically safe spaces for all nursing encounters by recognizing the widespread impact of prior trauma and its potential symptoms and working to prevent re-traumatization.

- To help foster trust and establish a therapeutic relationship with TNGE clients, nurses can convey empathy by acknowledging an understanding of challenges TNGE people experience in health care environments, and they should respond accordingly by explaining what the nurse will do to address any challenge or structural issue that may hinder the delivery of gender-affirming nursing care.

- Nurses should mirror the language used by TNGE clients; ask for clarification if clients use unfamiliar language to describe some aspect of their identity, anatomy, or health-related behavior; and obtain consent and provide anticipatory guidance before beginning the physical assessment and throughout the care encounter.

DISCLOSURES

Dr Cicero was supported by a grant from the Alzheimer's Association, United States (23AARGD-NTF-1028973). The statements in this article are solely the responsibility of the author and do not necessarily represent the views of the Alzheimer's Association.

REFERENCES

1. Coleman E, Radix AE, Bouman WP, et al. Standards of care for the health of transgender and gender diverse people, version 8. Int J Transgend Health 2022; 23(sup 1):S1–259.
2. Butler J. Gender Trouble, Feminism and the Subversion of Identity. New York, NY: Routledge; 1990.
3. Sevelius J. Gender affirmation: A framework for conceptualizing risk behavior among transgender women of color. Sex Roles 2013;68(11–12):675–89.
4. Reisner SL, Radix A, Deutsch MB. Integrated and gender-affirming transgender clinical care and research. J Acquir Immune Defic Syndr 2016;72:S235–42.
5. Hughes TL, Jackman K, Dorsen C, et al. How can the nursing profession help reduce sexual and gender minority related health disparities: Recommendations from the National Nursing LGBTQ Health Summit. Nurs Outlook 2022;70(3): 513–24.
6. Jones JM. U.S. LGBT identification steady at 7.2%. Gallup. Updated February 22, 2023. Accessed August 1, 2023. Available at: https://news.gallup.com/poll/470708/lgbt-identification-steady.aspx.
7. Myers A. Trans-formations. How evolving trans terminology around sex and gender can help us all. 2018. Available at: https://slate.com/human-interest/2018/05/trans-terminologys-constant-evolution-is-good-for-everyone.html Accessed August 15, 2023.
8. Cicero EC, Lunn MR, Obedin-Maliver J, et al. Acceptability of biospecimen collection among sexual and/or gender minority adults in the United States. Ann LGBTQ Public Popul Health 2023. https://doi.org/10.1891/LGBTQ-2022-0021.
9. Beischel WJ, Gauvin SEM, van Anders SM. "A little shiny gender breakthrough": Community understandings of gender euphoria. Int J Transgend Health 2022; 23(3):274–94.
10. Beemyn G. A presence in the past: A transgender historiography. J Womens Hist 2013;25(4):113–21.
11. O'Sullivan S. The colonial project of gender (and everything else). Genealogy 2021;5(3):67.
12. McClintock A. Imperial Leather Race, Gender, and Sexuality in the Colonial Contest. New York, NY: Routledge; 2013.

13. Ashley F., Buchanan B., The anti-trans panic is rooted in white supremacist ideology. Truthout. 2023. Available at: https://truthout.org/articles/the-anti-trans-panic-is-rooted-in-white-supremacist-ideology/. Accessed August 1, 2023.

14. Carrier L, Dame J, Lane J. Two-Spirit identity and Indigenous conceptualization of gender and sexuality: Implications for nursing practice. Creativ Nurs 2020;26(2): 96–100.

15. Dutta A. Elsewheres in queer Hindutva: A Hijra case study. Fem Rev 2023;133(1): 11–25.

16. Soldatic K, Briskman L, Trewlynn W, et al. Social and emotional wellbeing of indigenous gender and sexuality diverse youth: Mapping the evidence. Cult Health Sex 2022;24(4):564–82.

17. Puckett JA, Tornello S, Mustanski B, et al. Gender variations, generational effects, and mental health of transgender people in relation to timing and status of gender identity milestones. Psychol Sex Orientat Gend Divers 2022;9(2):165–78.

18. Gamarel KE, Jadwin-Cakmak L, King WM, et al. Improving access to legal gender affirmation for transgender women involved in the criminal–legal system. J Correct Health Care 2023;29(1):12–5.

19. Smart BD, Mann-Jackson L, Alonzo J, et al. Transgender women of color in the U.S. South: A qualitative study of social determinants of health and healthcare perspectives. Int J Transgend Health 2022/04/03 2022;23(1–2):164–77.

20. James SE, Herman JL, Rankin S, et al. The report of the 2015 U.S. Transgender survey. National Center for Transgender Equality; 2016. Available at: https://transequality.org/sites/default/files/docs/usts/USTS-Full-Report-Dec17.pdf. Accessed August 1, 2023.

21. White Hughto JM, Reisner SL, Pachankis JE. Transgender stigma and health: A critical review of stigma determinants, mechanisms, and interventions. Soc Sci Med 2015;147:222–31.

22. Mumford K, Fraser L, Knudson G. What the past suggests about when a diagnostic label is oppressive. AMA J Ethics 2023;25(6):446–51.

23. World Health Organization. Gender incongruence and transgender health in the ICD https://www.who.int/standards/classifications/frequently-asked-questions/gender-incongruence-and-transgender-health-in-the-icd. Accessed July 28, 2023.

24. Human Rights Campaign. Fatal violence against the transgender and gender non-conforming community in 2021 Available at: https://www.hrc.org/resources/fatal-violence-against-the-transgender-and-gender-non-conforming-community-in-2021. Accessed August 1, 2023.

25. Hendricks ML, Testa RJ. A conceptual framework for clinical work with transgender and gender nonconforming clients: An adaptation of the Minority Stress Model. Prof Psychol Res Pract 2012;43(5):460–7.

26. Cicero EC, Reisner SL, Silva SG, et al. Health care experiences of transgender adults: An integrated mixed research literature review. ANS Adv Nurs Sci 2019; 42(2):123–38.

27. Miller LR, Grollman EA. The social costs of gender nonconformity for transgender adults: Implications for discrimination and health. Sociol Forum 2015;30(3): 809–31.

28. Hatzenbuehler ML, Phelan JC, Link BG. Stigma as a fundamental cause of population health inequalities. Am J Public Health 2013;103(5):813–21.

29. Suess Schwend A. Trans health care from a depathologization and human rights perspective. Publ Health Rev 2020;41(1):3.

30. Badgett M, Choi SK, Wilson BD. LGBT poverty in the United States: a study of differences between sexual orientation and gender identity groups. The Williams Institute; 2019. Available at: https://williamsinstitute.law.ucla.edu/wp-content/uploads/National-LGBT-Poverty-Oct-2019.pdf. Accessed August 1, 2023.

31. Downing J, Lawley KA, McDowell A. Prevalence of private and public health insurance among transgender and gender diverse adults. Med Care 2022;60(4):311–5.

32. Romero AP, Goldberg SK, Vasquez LA. LGBT people and housing affordability, discrimination, and homelessness. The Williams Institute; 2020. Available at: https://williamsinstitute.law.ucla.edu/wp-content/uploads/LGBT-Housing-Apr-2020.pdf. Accessed August 1, 2023.

33. Cicero EC, Reisner S, Merwin E, et al. The health status of transgender and gender nonbinary adults in the United States. PLoS One 2020;15(2):e0228765.

34. Downing JM, Przedworski JM. Health of transgender adults in the U.S., 2014-2016. Am J Prev Med 2018;55(3):336–44.

35. Dragon C, Guerino P, Ewald E, et al. Transgender Medicare beneficiaries and chronic conditions: Exploring fee-for-service claims data. LGBT Health 2017;4(6):404–11.

36. Juster R-P, McEwen BS, Lupien SJ. Allostatic load biomarkers of chronic stress and impact on health and cognition. Neurosci Biobehav Rev 2010;35(1):2–16.

37. Velasco RAF, Reed SM. Nursing, social justice, and health inequities: A critical analysis of the theory of emancipatory nursing praxis. ANS Adv Nurs Sci 2023;46(3):249–64.

38. Sallans RK. Lessons from a transgender patient for health care professionals. AMA J Ethics 2016;18(11):1139–46.

39. Kodadek LM, Peterson S, Shields RY, et al. Collecting sexual orientation and gender identity information in the emergency department: The divide between patient and provider perspectives. Emerg Med J 2019;36(3):136–41.

40. Maragh-Bass AC, Torain M, Adler R, et al. Is it okay to ask: Transgender patient perspectives on sexual orientation and gender identity collection in healthcare. Acad Emerg Med 2017;24(6):655–67.

41. Ruben MA, Blosnich JR, Dichter ME, et al. Will veterans answer sexual orientation and gender identity questions? Med Care 2017;55:S85–9.

42. Cahill S, Singal R, Grasso C, et al. Do ask, do tell: High levels of acceptability by patients of routine collection of sexual orientation and gender identity data in four diverse American community health centers. PLoS One 2014;9(9):e107104.

43. Wesley C, Manaoat Van C, Mossburg SE. Patient safety concerns and the LGBTQ+ population. Agency for Healthcare Research and Quality. 2023, Available at: https://psnet.ahrq.gov/perspective/patient-safety-concerns-and-lgbtq-population. Accessed August 1, 2023.

44. National LGBT Health Education Center. Taking routine histories of sexual health: a system-wide approach for health centers. Fenway Health; 2015. Available at: https://lgbtqiahealtheducation.org/wp-content/uploads/COM-827-sexual-history_toolkit_2015.pdf. Accessed August 1, 2023.

45. Ragosta S, Obedin-Maliver J, Fix L, et al. From 'shark-week' to 'mangina': An analysis of words used by people of marginalized sexual orientations and/or gender identities to replace common sexual and reproductive health terms. Health Equity 2021;5(1):707–17.

46. McDowell M, Pardee DJ, Peitzmeier S, et al. Cervical cancer screening preferences among trans-masculine individuals: Patient-collected human

papillomavirus vaginal swabs versus provider-administered pap tests. LGBT Health 2017;4(4):252–9.

47. Reisner SL, Deutsch MB, Peitzmeier SM, et al. Test performance and acceptability of self-versus provider-collected swabs for high-risk HPV DNA testing in female-to-male trans masculine patients. PLoS One 2018;13(3):e0190172.

48. Cicero EC, Black BP. "I was a spectacle a freak show at the circus": A transgender person's ED experience and implications for nursing practice. J Emerg Nurs 2016;42(1):25–30.

49. Pulice-Farrow L, Lindley L, Gonzalez KA. "Wait, what is that? A man or woman or what?": Trans microaggressions from gynecological healthcare providers. Sex Res Soc Pol 2022;19(4):1549–60.

50. Kronk CA, Everhart AR, Ashley F, et al. Transgender data collection in the electronic health record: Current concepts and issues. J Am Med Inf Assoc 2021; 29(2):271–84.

51. Grasso C, Goldhammer H, Thompson J, et al. Optimizing gender-affirming medical care through anatomical inventories, clinical decision support, and population health management in electronic health record systems. J Am Med Inf Assoc 2021;28(11):2531–5.

52. Alpert AB, Mehringer JE, Orta SJ, et al. Experiences of transgender people reviewing their electronic health records, a qualitative study. J Gen Intern Med 2022;38(4):970–7.

53. Chang BL, Sayyed AA, Haffner ZK, et al. Perioperative misgendering experiences in patients undergoing gender-affirming surgery: A call for a gender-inclusive healthcare environment. Eur J Plast Surg 2023;1–9.

54. The Joint Commission. What are the key elements organizations need to understand regarding the use of two patient identifiers prior to providing care, treatment or services? Updated August 29, 2022, https://www.jointcommission.org/standards/standard-faqs/home-care/national-patient-safety-goals-npsg/00000 1545/#:~:text=Acceptable%20identifiers%20may%20be%20the,of%20a% 20unique%20patient%20identifier. Accessed August 1, 2023.

55. Hagen DB, Galupo MP. Trans* individuals' experiences of gendered language with health care providers: Recommendations for practitioners. Int J Transgenderism 2014;15(1):16–34.

56. Lambda Legal. Creating equal access to quality health care for transgender patients: transgender affirming hospital policies. 2013. https://legacy.lambdalegal.org/publications/fs_transgender-affirming-hospital-policies. Accessed August 1, 2023.

57. American Nurses Association. Code of Ethics for nurses with interpretive statements. 2nd ed. American Nurses Association; 2015:64 https://www.nursingworld.org/practice-policy/nursing-excellence/ethics/code-of-ethics-for-nurses/. Accessed August 1, 2023.

58. Cicero EC. Anti-transgender legislation and gender-affirming care bans: Are position statements without subsequent nursing action the equivalent of thoughts and prayers? Nurs Outlook 2023;71(4). online.

59.. Eliason MJ, Chinn PL. LGBTQ Cultures: What Health Care Professionals Need to Know, . About Sexual and Gender Diversity. 3rd edition. Philadelphia, PA: Lippincott Williams & Wilkins; 2017.

60. Dillard-Wright J, Shields-Haas V. Nursing with the people: Reimagining futures for nursing. ANS Adv Nurs Sci 2021;44(3):195–209.

61. Americans continue to rank nurses most honest and ethical professionals. Press release. ANA Enterprise; Janurary 10, 2023 https://www.nursingworld.org/news/

news-releases/2022-news-releases/americans-continue-to-rank-nurses-most-ho nest-and-ethical-professionals/. Accessed August 1, 2023.

62. Ducar D. The urgent need for authentic leadership and allyship in health care. J Cont Educ Nurs 2023;54(5):201–3.

63. Perron A, Rudge T, Gagnon M. Towards an "Ethics of Discomfort" in Nursing: Parrhesia as Fearless Speech. In: Philosophies and Practices of Emancipatory Nursing: Social Justice as Praxis. New York, NY: Routledge; 2014. p. 39–50.

64. Anwar A, Abid G, Waqas A. Authentic leadership and creativity: Moderated meditation model of resilience and hope in the health sector. Eur J Investig Health Psychol Educ 2020;10(1):18–29.

A Cultural Humility Approach to Inclusive and Equitable Nursing Care

Linda Johanson, EdD, MS(n), RN[a],
Patti P. Urso, PhD, APRN, ANP-BC, FNP, CNE[b],
Mary A. Bemker, PhD, PsyS, CNE, RN[b],
Debra Sullivan, PhD, MSN, RN, CNE, COI[b,*]

KEYWORDS

- Cultural humility • Cultural competence • Nursing education
- Nursing health care delivery • Nursing care

KEY POINTS

- US population is changing rapidly, and nurses must be prepared to offer inclusive and equitable nursing care.
- Cultural humility goes beyond cultural competence as a perpetual learning role from the individual patients who are the experts of their culture.
- Bedside nurses can practice cultural humility to those with differing backgrounds by including active listening, being humble, having self-awareness, and practicing self-reflection as it is a lifelong process.

INTRODUCTION

An essential role of nurses has always been to help people live their healthiest life possible, which can only be achieved through health equity.[1] The nursing workforce must provide inclusive, equitable, and diverse care.[2] Despite efforts to practice cultural competency as taught historically in nursing curriculums, disparities in health equity remain.[3] The expectation that one could be taught to be competent in all cultures is an impossible expectation. Cultural humility is a move forward that can better prepare nurses for culturally appropriate care.[4] The concept of cultural humility goes beyond ethnic or racial differences as it promotes consideration of a person's culture from the individual's view while developing mutually respectful and dynamic

[a] Walden University, College of Nursing, 100 Washington Avenue South, Suite 1210, Minneapolis, MN 55401, USA; [b] Walden University College of Nursing, 100 Washington Avenue South, Suite 900, Minneapolis, MN 55401, USA
* Corresponding author.
E-mail address: debra.sullivan@mail.waldenu.edu

partnerships.[5] Cultural humility includes active listening to those with differing backgrounds, self-awareness, and self-reflection as it is a lifelong process.[3] The following narrative review will offer insight into how to provide inclusive and equitable nursing care by using concepts provided by cultural humility.

BACKGROUND

The US population is changing rapidly. The most significant population decrease was seen in the white (non-Hispanic) group, from 63.8% in 2010 to 59.3% in 2021, whereas the Hispanic/Latino group increased the most from 2.5% to 18.9%.[6] The nursing workforce increased in racial and ethnic diversity in 2020, but not as fast as the population: 69% are white, 12% Black/African American, 9.1 Asian, with only 7.4% are Hispanic.[1] By 2030, the nursing workforce will be challenged to create health equity with an even more diverse population.[1] Although these demographics change in the United States, learning to apply cultural humility can shape nursing attitudes and expand intercultural understanding.[7]

Cultural humility is defined nicely in a concept analysis by Foronda and colleagues[8] "In a multicultural world where power imbalances exist, cultural humility is a process of openness, self-awareness, being egoless, and incorporating self-reflection and critique after willingly interacting with diverse individuals. The results of achieving cultural humility are mutual empowerment, respect, partnerships, optimal care, and lifelong learning."[(p 4)] In their analysis, Foronda and colleagues[8] recommend that instead of memorizing attributes of various cultures, one should attempt to change their perspectives and accept cultural humility as a way of life. It means being constantly aware of power imbalances and being humble in all interactions with everyone, including personal and professional encounters.[8] An essential element to note is that culture encompasses not only ethnic and racial culture but also social diversity such as socioeconomic status, individual ranks in different walks of life, and differences in gender, lesbian, gay, bisexual, and transgender community.[8]

Melanie Tervalon and Jann Murray-Garcia developed the term cultural humility in 1998 to address inequities noted in health care delivery.[9] This concept comprised three elements: (1) cultural humility focused on a lifelong commitment to openness and self-evaluation, (2) aspiring to correct power imbalances, being egoless, and (3) collaborating with diverse individuals.[5,8] However, there are many different interpretations and understandings of cultural humility.

When looking at these three elements of cultural humility, it is crucial to recognize that one is never complete with self-reflection and personal growth. One must also acknowledge that everyone has a lived experience that promotes their worth as individuals and to society. In response, the power imbalance is positively impacted. As a result, individuals commit to making positive changes toward rectifying these imbalances individually and as part of a community.[10]

Similar to the Tervalon and Murray-Garcia[5] conceptualization, Chang and colleagues[4] address cultural humility using the QIAN model. QIAN, or humbleness in Chinese, compiles the elements of cultural humility and health care education. Self-questioning (Q), bidirectional cultural emersion (I), active listening (A), and negotiation (N) are the components of this model.

Foronda and colleagues[8] expanded the understanding of the term cultural humility through concept analysis. In addition to ethnic differences, cultural humility can apply to such areas as geographic locale, sexual preferences, socioeconomic divergence, and interprofessional roles and conceptualization. Specific attributes supporting cultural humility were openness, self-awareness, egoless, supportive interactions, and self-reflection—outcomes of such support mutual empowerment, partnerships, optimal care, and lifelong learning.

Nurses are challenged to overcome the precedents impacting injustice and inequality. Nurses must rise above any need to justify individual value at the expense of others and readily appreciate diverse perspectives and understanding. This practice enhances the overall profession and organization through increased inclusivity.[10] Otherwise, a psychologically safe place will not be fostered, and nurse retention will continue to be problematic for those who do not feel supported.[11]

Paradigm Shift from Cultural Competence to Cultural Humility

The concept of cultural competence includes a knowledge base of cultural beliefs, values, and practices that may impact patient care and the importance of providing culturally competent care to improve patient outcomes.[12] Cultural competency constructs involve the ability to navigate and understand diverse cultures, by developing cultural awareness, cultural knowledge, cultural skill, cultural encounters, and cultural desire which is particularly important when caring for patients from various backgrounds.[13] Being cultural competent is a worthy aim for a nurse, but unattainable in a health care setting where patients present with a wide range of cultures and ethnicities. It is important to recognize that people carry within themselves a wealth of experiences and cultural identities that go beyond what can be learned from books or firsthand encounters. As such, it is crucial to move beyond the goal of cultural competence with the promotion of cultural humility.

Cultural humility is a relatively newer concept that has gained recognition in nursing. It emphasizes ongoing self-reflection and a willingness to learn from patients, recognizing that health care providers may not fully understand the depth of each patient's cultural background.[12] It encompasses the acquisition of skills and awareness necessary to provide effective care and establish meaningful connections with patients from diverse cultural backgrounds. Cultural humility, in the context of nursing, is about acknowledging our own limitations and actively engaging in self-reflection regarding our personal cultural backgrounds, life experiences, individual identities, and ongoing learning about the experiences of others, particularly our patients.[14] Developing a culture that values and prioritizes the continual learning about diverse cultures, without elevating one above the others, fosters an inclusive and welcoming environment for all patients. In an ideal nursing environment, if every nurse would actively listen to patients and seek to learn about their unique cultural backgrounds, such as being from a culture different from the dominant one, is not viewed as inferior or less significant. This approach confronts the disparities that diverse populations experience in health care and ensures that every patient receives respectful and culturally appropriate care, ultimately enhancing the quality of health care delivery.[15]

LITERATURE REVIEW OF CULTURAL HUMILITY

Effective educational programs that embrace cultural humility practices and use valid measurement tools promote culturally humble education and nursing care. This practice allows nursing educators, students, and graduates to have the necessary tools to direct and evaluate their knowledge and attitudes that promote culturally humble health care delivery. As the US population continues to experience sociodemographic shifts, it is important that nurses are prepared to provide adequate care for all.[15,16]

Cultural humility has also been shown to promote student satisfaction with nurses providing education. A direct correlation between the student's perception of the nursing faculty's utilization of cultural humility and student approval of the faculty has been noted.[17,18]

If nurses are to provide quality care, it is essential for nurses to be expected to care for diverse populations. To provide a healthy work environment, educators and practicing nurses must model appropriate behaviors and increase cultural understanding and experiences through a more comprehensive inclusion of aspects of various cultures in their education, employment orientation, and continuing education.[7,16,19,20] Educators, leadership, and bedside nurses can decrease bias and support these inclusive environments. In turn, this focus can increase retention.[20] It has been noted that nursing students and practicing nurses' ability to adjust to the educational and work norms are enhanced when cultural humility is at the fore.[21,22]

Cultural humility is essential for nurse educators to improve faculty–student relationships and those interactions between nurses and patients. Promoting faculty and students' awareness of their own personal perspectives on cultural humility and biases implicit and explicit within that framework increases a connection between individuals. This connection serves as a foundation in enabling educators, students, and graduates to direct and evaluate attitudes that promote culturally humble health care delivery.[16] Cultural humility serves as a platform to promote student satisfaction with their faculty members. A direct correlation between a student's perception of nursing faculty demonstrating cultural humility and student approval of the instructor has been noted.[17]

When addressing the unique qualities of individuals, it is important to listen and understand where the student or patient is coming from on their life journey. We are all unique within our culture, gender, geographic region, and so forth. By looking at individuals as unique within various classes or categories, we are able to join specifically with that individual instead of treating the individual as a "number" among a defined group. The need for cultural infusion content and practice continues to be paramount.[23]

Implicit biases are of particular concern when relating with others who share differences from our own. Cultural humility serves as a means of uncovering such beliefs that are often deeply embedded and can be subconscious.[24] This dynamic is of particular concern among health care professionals,[24–26] It needs to be addressed by nurses in all environments so that they can continue to address any such biases in relation to students, patients, and coworkers. Marginalized ideas related to cultural differences can result in misinterpretations, conflicts, and damaged relationships.[27] A more respectful engagement and relationship emerges by addressing perceptions that drive behavior and are often unnoticed.[25]

CASE STUDY

When student nurses are challenged to create a plan of care for a clinical patient, they are to consider holistic health. The physical diagnosis is researched, what mental stresses might be interrelated, spiritual components, and environmental and family dynamics. Consider this very plausible case:

Josie, an eager, competent student, has received an assignment to care for a newly diagnosed patient diagnosed with diabetes man, age 30, of Mexican heritage, who entered the medical center through the emergency department (ED) in ketoacidosis. After treatment in the ED, this patient has been transferred to the medical unit for further stabilization. This note is the only information available to Josie, the student nurse, to begin crafting a care plan. On preconference meeting with the instructor, the student shares the plan is to concentrate on patient teaching now that the client has stabilized. She has proudly researched information on the care of the Hispanic patient from her textbook and will include members of what she anticipates will be a large family. She has learned some Spanish words and has downloaded an application to her phone with Spanish health translation. The instructor encourages her in her preparation toward cultural care. However, when the student meets the client, she finds he is sharing quiet words with his same-sex spouse. He does not know Spanish, as he was raised in the United States. He is employed as a pharmacist and has a PhD. Suddenly, the student and instructor are very aware that they have stereotyped the patient based on preconceived notions of the Hispanic culture, and the drafted care plan will not be useful.

Jordan, a different student nurse, is presented with the same scenario, but Jordan has attended online nursing courses where the concepts of cultural humility were promoted in an inclusive learning environment. Five attributes of cultural humility were stressed throughout the curriculum: openness, self-awareness, being egoless, supportive interactions, and self-reflection.[28] Following is an example of a nursing care plan developed by Jordan using cultural humility as a framework.

- Assess the patient's level of openness to learning about diabetes management and his cultural beliefs and practices regarding health and illness.
- Demonstrate self-awareness of one's own biases, assumptions, and stereotypes about diabetes and Mexican culture, and avoid imposing one's own values or judgments on the patient.
- Be egoless and respectful of the patient's autonomy, dignity, and preferences, and acknowledge the power imbalance that may exist between the nurse and the patient.
- Provide supportive interactions that foster trust, rapport, and collaboration with the patient, his family, and other members of the health care team.
- Engage in self-reflection and seek feedback from the patient, his family, and other cultural brokers on how to improve one's cultural humility and competence in providing culturally sensitive care.

When using cultural humility as an approach to nursing care, the patient will be part of the decision-making process, truly providing patient-centered care. Including cultural humility in nursing curricula can not only promote transcultural nursing care but also fosters an inclusive and psychologically safe learning environment.[20] Based on the importance of cultural humility being included in the learning environment, the following pilot study was conducted to assess the nurse faculty's knowledge level of cultural humility.

ONLINE NURSE FACULTY KNOWLEDGE OF CULTURAL HUMILITY: A PILOT STUDY

Bedside nurses are taught some aspects of cultural care in nursing school, but it may be ineffective due to stereotypical ways of teaching cultural competence. The authors of this article wanted to consider ways that the approach of cultural humility might be introduced as an alternative to the traditional approach in academic nursing programs; however, a first step would be to conduct an assessment. It seemed critical to know if instructors actually know about the concept of cultural humility and even if they possess the traits associated with cultural humility themselves. Do teachers already use this approach in the classroom? To assess the prevalence of cultural humility among online nurse educators the following pilot study was designed and implemented.

Design

The pilot study was a nonexperimental descriptive design. The instrument selected was the Foronda's Cultural Humility Scale.[29] This tool was selected because it measures with high reliability and validity of the construct being studied.

Instrument

Permission to use the Foronda's Cultural Humility Scale was granted from the developer, who emailed the research team the instrument and the interpretation guide. The initial version of this instrument was determined to be reliable, with all items rated 0.83 or higher on factor analysis and valid with a score of Cronbach's alpha 0.85.[29] The team elected to use the revised version of the scale, which does not yet have completed psychometrics for the pilot. It is like the original but has four additional items, which the research team believed strengthened the validity of the tool.

The instrument consists of items constructed to reflect key constructs in cultural humility. Each of the 23 items is followed by a 5-point Likert scale in which respondents rate themselves as either never or rarely displaying that attribute (1 point), once in a while (2 points), sometimes (3 points), usually (4 points), or all the time (5 points). The items are summed to generate the score as follows (**Table 1**).

Ethics

The research was approved by the Institutional Review Board (IRB) of the institution where members are employed as nurse educators. All members of the research team have completed the Collaborative Institutional Training Initiative (CITI) training. A consent form was distributed for participants to read and agree to before joining the study.

Sampling

The sample was taken from the institution's Participant Pool. The Participant Pool at this institution is a Web site accessible by students and faculty who want to volunteer to participant in a research study. Current research studies are listed in the Participant Pool and the volunteer may access an invitation to participate in the research study. In addition, an invitation was distributed through departmental supervisors to all full- and part-time faculty who teach in the College of Nursing. The setting is an accredited online university with nursing programs in BSN completion, several Masters in Nursing specialties, including several nurse practitioner programs, and DNP/PhD programs of study. The invitation to the survey included a link to the online instrument and took approximately 5 minutes for participants to complete.

Table 1 Foronda's cultural humility interpretation guide (revised)	
Scores	**Category**
Scores 23–46	Rarely culturally humble
Scores 47–91	Sometimes culturally humble
Scores 92–103	Usually culturally humble
Score of 104–115	Habitually culturally humble

Findings

The survey was available for 2 weeks following the invitation. Sixty invitations were sent, and twenty-eight individuals responded. Twenty-five respondents were female and three were male. Sixteen possessed doctorates in nursing and ten non-nursing doctorates. There was one, each with a BSN and MSN.

Most respondents reported that the concept of cultural humility was part of the on-line courses that they had taught in the past. Nine indicated this concept was inte-grated into one course, and ten indicated that it was present in more than one course. Eight indicated they had taught courses in which cultural humility was not a part, and one had taught a course dedicated to the concept.

Findings from the survey indicated that most instructors displayed at least some cultural humility (**Table 2**). Only one participant was rated rarely culturally humble, and most were rated either sometimes or habitually culturally humble.

DISCUSSION

The research team recommends securing the psychometrics for the revised version of Foronda's Cultural Humility Scale and enlarging the participant pool by seeking collab-oration with other nursing programs. The online version of the instrument should be amended so that participants will receive an automatic score after completing the sur-vey. Further data analysis should be conducted with a larger sample to discern if there are any correlations between demographic data and cultural humility. The team would also like to add a qualitative component to the study by selecting respondents who scored as habitually culturally humble to describe how they perceived that trait emerged and how it can be used effectively in nursing education.

Based on these findings, that most instructors displayed at least some cultural hu-mility, it would be interesting to know if bedside nurses who graduated from online nursing programs feel that they practice cultural humility. The revised Foronda's Cul-tural Humility Scale with a qualitative component could be used to make this assess-ment and then compare the results to this study. It could also bring awareness of the components of cultural humility to bedside nurses.

IMPLICATIONS

The nursing profession requires care and compassion. From the beginning of a nurse's education, nurses have been taught to take into account the patient culture as a guide for nursing care. This attitude extrapolates to nursing education. However, the emphasis has been on cultural competence and lays on the nurse's shoulder the inherent responsibility to learn the patient's culture. In nursing education, understand-ing the student's culture is theoretically emphasized; however, in practice, the

Table 2 Findings from pilot study	
Category	Number of Participants in the Category
Rarely culturally humble	1
Sometimes culturally humble	12
Usually culturally humble	5
Habitually culturally humble	10

transmission of the traditions in nursing education has prevailed, often alienating rather than attracting individuals that will diversify the workforce. By contrast, cultural humility requires that the nurse search and be guided by the individual recipient of the care and takes away the role of the expert from the nursing profession. The nurse will guide the process, but the individual, be it a patient, nurse, or student is the expert.

Cultural competence can refer to the accumulated knowledge gained based on information collected from many individuals reading assumptions to the whole group. Paradoxically, gaining knowledge about culture should not be a static end but, instead, an ongoing process that will only be gained through cultural humility, allowing the professional to be in a perpetual learning role from the individuals who are the expert of their culture. These two approaches to learning about culture are often confused.

IMPLICATIONS FOR NURSE EDUCATORS

This pilot study has implications for the online instructor. First and foremost, it increases the awareness of the instructor's knowledge deficit on the topic. Some participants expressed a lack of familiarity with the central concepts of cultural humility and asked for a definition. These insights demonstrate a lack of knowledge on the topic and the need to educate online instructors about this important approach that leads to a true understanding of nurses' and students' learning need. Professional development opportunities for nurses, coupled with online instruction, should focus on the ongoing journey of fostering cultural humility via self-reflective exercises and honing communication skills. This approach nurtures a sincere curiosity about each student's individual cultural heritage.

Further research should be expanded to understand how being culturally humble can be implemented in nursing and the nursing curricula that includes development and teaching modalities to address the social determinants of health. The Foronda's Cultural Humility Scale measurements focused on self-assessment at the moment in time as a point of feedback for the participant.[29] Still, it can be suggested that it be kept as a tool for lifelong learning, discovery, and critical self-analysis for the purpose of growth. The outcome of this analysis invariably leads toward greater genuineness and respect. Being able to reach into the community will require these values in significant quantities to gain trust from individuals and communities.

RECOMMENDATIONS FOR NURSE EDUCATORS

Educating individuals on the concept of cultural humility in the process of understanding another culture necessitates an awareness of one's own personal biases. This journey of self-awareness is not a simple one, as it requires individuals to confront their implicit and explicit biases. In the context of education, students can benefit from various exercises designed to help them recognize and reflect on their biases. Journaling is a powerful tool in this process, encouraging students to engage in focused introspection with specific prompts. Essential questions such as "Why do I feel negative feelings about?" or "What if this person was more like me?" can guide them in exploring the origins of their biases and how their past experiences contribute to these feelings. Removing self-judgment is crucial because it allows students to delve deeper into understanding themselves and their biases, ultimately facilitating their journey toward cultural humility. Teaching students how to practice this self-reflection is an essential first step in promoting cultural competence.

In the Cultural Humility Toolkit discussed by Foronda and colleagues,[28] recommendations for the classroom include examining the environment, curriculum, teaching materials, and teaching methods, to be sure instruction is provided in a diverse environment. Also, to include cultural humility concepts in simulation and debriefing. Another idea is to offer study abroad opportunities.

Another effective classroom strategy for fostering cultural humility is group sharing. Encouraging students to share their reflections and experiences in a supportive group setting can be immensely beneficial. To facilitate this, sections of the students' journals can be submitted to the instructor, who can then share them anonymously within the group. Ground rules of respect and open-mindedness should serve as guiding principles during these discussions, creating a safe space for students to express their thoughts and feelings without fear of judgment.

Role playing in a simulation is yet another valuable tool for promoting cultural humility. By engaging in role-play exercises, students can immerse themselves in different cultural scenarios. An impromptu interview as a role-play activity students can practice defining the differences between leading questions and open questions and how to use them effectively. Through role play, students can gain hands-on experience in navigating cultural encounters and learning to ask open-ended, culturally sensitive questions, thus promoting a deeper understanding of diverse perspectives and backgrounds. These strategies collectively contribute to the development of cultural humility, a fundamental skill in our increasingly interconnected world.

Games offer different approaches to exploring cultures and promoting cultural humility indirectly by encouraging players to engage with diverse worlds, stories, and characters. Although they may not explicitly teach the concept, they can help players develop empathy and a more open-minded attitude toward cultural differences. Although there may not be specific video games designed explicitly to teach cultural humility, some games can indirectly promote empathy, tolerance, and cross-cultural understanding. You can also adapt popular board games. Foronda and colleagues[28] discussed games such as monopoly; changing the rules to simulate real situations, such as poverty and stigma.

Online instruction can seem impersonal and distant to some of those engaged; however, the injection of cultural humility as an approach to online teaching can be a game changer when it comes to warming up the online classroom. Future research is needed on how approaches rooted in cultural humility can be a tool for engaging students and modeling a lifelong bridge to differences.

RECOMMENDATIONS FOR THE BEDSIDE NURSE

Patient-centeredness is caring for the whole person and is the foundation of nursing care. The bedside nurse partners with the patient to consider the individual's health care needs in making health care decisions within the context of the patient's emotional, mental, spiritual, social, and financial perspectives. However, this ideal may not be effectively practiced by nurses as studies have revealed that 80% of nurses exhibit racial biases, and 90% have shown classist biases.[15] When looking at data related to US health care providers, nearly 17% were not born in the United States, and nearly 5% are noncitizens.[30] It is imperative that nurses and others with who we work feel welcome. Differences need to be celebrated and integrated into practice as much as possible. Active listening, acceptance of other cultures and opinions, and self-reflection on one's beliefs and relationships with others assist in supporting such.[5]

Nurses are human and human nature has an innate bias, both explicit and implicit, which can cause unintended discrimination as a consequence. Cultural humility goes beyond cultural competency and uncovers deeply embedded beliefs and addresses bias.[24] Cultural humility promotes self-reflection, which can help with recognizing bias. It also promotes active listening with respectful therapeutic communication, which can reveal social history and help tailor care to include social determinants of health such as culture, support system, access to food, living environment, work history, and transportation.

Nurses can practice cultural humility by having an open mind, being self-aware, being egoless (humble), having supportive interactions (active listening), and being self-reflective.[8] Foronda and colleagues[8] further states that "the results of achieving cultural humility are mutual empowerment, respect, partnerships, optimal care, and life-long learning."[(p4)]

SUMMARY

Cultural competency has been part of the nursing curriculum and part of nursing care for decades; however, we still see health disparities. Cultural humility transcends cultural competency with self-awareness and respecting the patient's perspective and views in a dynamic relationship. There is interest and some adoption of the concepts of cultural humility in nursing education; however, it is not well studied in nurses, nursing students, or online or traditional nursing education. A pilot study was completed to assess the prevalence of cultural humility among online nurse educators. Findings from the survey indicated that most instructors displayed at least some cultural humility. Still, a larger study would offer more insight into the need for more integration of cultural humility concepts. This research and narrative review have implications for bedside nurses, nursing students, and the online instructor to increase awareness on the topic and a need to integrate concepts of cultural humility into the practice of bedside nurses. Recommendations are offered for incorporating the principles of cultural humility into the roles of both nurse educators and bedside nurse.

CLINICS CARE POINTS

- Bedside nurses who practice cultural humility can promote inclusive and equitable nursing care.
- Cultural humility goes beyond cultural competency, offering a perpetual learning role from the patients they care for.
- Cultural humility is not well understood or practiced by nursing faculty, nursing students, or practicing nursing.
- Cultural humility should be part of a nursing curriculum and as a nurse competency while practicing providing patient-centered care.

DISCLOSURE

The authors have nothing to disclose.

REFERENCES

1. Flaubert JL, Le Menestrel S, Williams DR, et al, editors. National Academies of Sciences, Engineering, and Medicine; National Academy of Medicine; Committee on the Future of Nursing 2020–2030. The future of nursing 2020-2030: charting a path to achieve health equity. Washington (DC): National Academies Press

(US); 2021. Available at: http://www.ncbi.nlm.nih.gov/books/NBK573914/. Accessed August 4, 2023.

2. American Association of Colleges of Nursing. The essentials: core competencies for professional nursing education. 2021. Available at: https://www.aacnnursing.org/Portals/0/PDFs/Publications/Essentials-2021.pdf. Accessed August 4, 2023.

3. Isaacson M. Clarifying concepts: cultural humility or competency. J Prof Nurs 2014;30(3):251–8.

4. Chang ES, Simon M, Dong X. Integrating cultural humility into health care professional education and training. Adv Health Sci Educ 2012;17(2):269–78.

5. Tervalon M, Murray-García J. Cultural humility versus cultural competence: a critical distinction in defining physician training outcomes in multicultural education. J Health Care Poor Underserved 1998;9(2):117–25.

6. US population by year, race, age, ethnicity, & more. USAFacts. Available at: https://usafacts.org/data/topics/people-society/population-and-demographics/our-changing-population/. Published August 4, 2023. Accessed August 4, 2023.

7. Hughes V, Delva S, Nkimbeng M, et al. Not missing the opportunity: Strategies to promote cultural humility among future nursing faculty. J Prof Nurs 2020;36(1): 28–33.

8. Foronda C, Baptiste DL, Reinholdt MM, et al. Cultural humility: a concept analysis. J Transcult Nurs 2016;27(3):210–7.

9. Project READY: Reimagining Equity & Access for Diverse Youth – A free online professional development curriculum. Available at: https://ready.web.unc.edu/. Accessed August 4, 2023.

10. Gallegos JL, Karagory PM. Social justice and the nurse leader. In: Advancing Organizations Through Exemplary Nursing Leadership. DESTech Publications.

11. White BJ, Fulton JS. Common experiences of African American nursing students: an integrative review. Nurs Educ Perspect 2015;36(3):167–76.

12. Nolan TS, Alston A, Choto R, et al. Cultural humility. Clin J Oncol Nurs 2021; 25(5):3–9.

13. Campinha-Bacote Josepha. Coming to know cultural competence: an evolutionary process. Int J Hum Caring 2011;15(3):42–8.

14. Greene-Moton E, Minkler M. Cultural competence or cultural humility? moving beyond the debate. Health Promot Pract 2020;21(1):142–5.

15. Nolan TS, Alston A, Choto R, et al. Cultural humility: retraining and retooling nurses to provide equitable cancer care. Clin J Oncol Nurs 2021;25(5):3–9.

16. Allwright K, Goldie C, Almost J, et al. Fostering positive spaces in public health using a cultural humility approach. Public Health Nurs Boston Mass 2019;36(4): 551–6.

17. Abdul-Raheem J. Cultural humility in nursing education. J Cult Divers 2018;25(2): 66–73.

18. Alpert A, Kamen C, Schabath MB, et al. What exactly are we measuring? evaluating sexual and gender minority cultural humility training for oncology care clinicians. J Clin Oncol 2020;38(23):2605–9.

19. Patallo BJ. The multicultural guidelines in practice: cultural humility in clinical training and supervision. Train Educ Prof Psychol 2019;13(3):227–32.

20. Smith A, Foronda C. Promoting cultural humility in nursing education through the use of ground rules. Nurs Educ Perspect 2021;42(2):117–9.

21. Englund H. The Relationship Between Marginality and Undergraduate Nursing Students. August 2017. https://twu-ir.tdl.org/bitstream/handle/11274/9331/2017EnglundOCR.pdf?sequence=3&isAllowed=y. Accessed August 5, 2023.

22. Iheduru-Anderson K, Shingles RR, Akanegbu C. Discourse of race and racism in nursing: An integrative review of literature - Iheduru-Anderson - 2021 - public health nursing - wiley online library. Public Health Nurs 2021;38(1):115–30.

23. Sellers WE, Kirven J. Exploring cultural humility and online programs: mid-career academics and changing times. Reflect Narrat Prof Help 2019;25(1):49–56.

24. FitzGerald C, Hurst S. Implicit bias in healthcare professionals: a systematic review. BMC Med Ethics 2017;18(1):19.

25. Markey K, Prosen M, Martin E, et al. Fostering an ethos of cultural humility development in nurturing inclusiveness and effective intercultural team working. J Nurs Manag 2021;29(8):2724–8.

26. Sprik P, Gentile D. Cultural humility: a way to reduce LGBTQ health disparities at the end of life. Am J Hosp Palliat Med 2020;37(6):404–8.

27. Kaihlanen AM, Hietapakka L, Heponiemi T. Increasing cultural awareness: qualitative study of nurses' perceptions about cultural competence training. BMC Nurs 2019;18(1):38.

28. Foronda C, Prather S, Baptiste DL, et al. Cultural humility toolkit. Nurse Educ 2022;47(5):267–71.

29. Foronda C, Porter A, Phitwong A. Psychometric testing of an instrument to measure cultural humility. J Transcult Nurs 2021;32(4):399–404.

30. Patel YM, Ly DP, Hicks T, et al. Proportion of non–US-born and noncitizen health care professionals in the United States in 2016. JAMA 2018;320(21):2265.

Promoting Health Equity Among Marginalized and Vulnerable Populations

Josepha Campinha-Bacote, PhD, MAR, PMHCNS-BC, CTN-A, FAAN, FTNSS,

KEYWORDS

- Cultural competemility • Health equity • Health inequities • Health disparities
- Vulnerable populations • Marginalized populations • Cultural humility
- Cultural competence

KEY POINTS

- The concept of culture and its relationships to health is critical to comprehend when rendering healthcare services to marginalized and vulnerable populations.
- Interactions reflecting implicit bias can result in lower quality care and perpetuate health disparities.
- Cultural humility and cultural competence must enter into a synergetic relationship.
- There is a need for structural competency among healthcare professionals in rendering care to vulnerable and marginalized populations.
- Promoting health equity among marginalized and vulnerable populations necessitates a full spectrum of outcomes spanning from downstream, midstream, and upstream approaches.

INTRODUCTION

In 2021, *The Future of Nursing 2020–2030: Charting a Path to Achieve Health Equity*,[1] *The Essentials: Core Competencies for Professional Nursing Education*,[2] and The International Council of Nurses Code of Ethics for Nurses[3] all called on nurses to advocate for equity and emphasize the role of nurses in promoting health equity. Moreover, Moss and Phillips[4] emphasized that social justice is a key aspect of health equity as well as a core concept of nursing ethics. The American Nurses Association defines social justice as "the analysis, critique, and change of social structures, policies, laws, customs, power, and privilege that disadvantage or harm vulnerable social groups through marginalization, exclusion, exploitation, and voicelessness."[5] (p63)

Equitable health outcomes are possible when actions are directed toward elimination of social inequalities that create disadvantages and limit the life chances including

Transcultural C.A.R.E, Associates, 11108 Huntwicke Place, Blue Ash, OH 45241, USA
E-mail address: meddir@aol.com

Nurs Clin N Am 59 (2024) 109–120
https://doi.org/10.1016/j.cnur.2023.11.009
0029-6465/24/© 2023 Elsevier Inc. All rights reserved.
nursing.theclinics.com

the health of certain population groups.[6,7] There are several terms that are used to describe these populations, which include disadvantaged, targeted, hard/difficult to reach, underserved, disenfranchised, disempowered, underprivileged, at-risk, high risk, vulnerable, and marginalized.[8] This article will focus on promoting health equity among marginalized and vulnerable populations.

VULNERABLE AND MARGINALIZED POPULATIONS

Waisel[9] defines vulnerable populations as groups who are at increased risk of receiving a disparity in medical care on the basis of financial circumstances or social characteristics such as age, race, gender, ethnicity, sexual orientation, spirituality, disability, or socioeconomic or insurance status. These characteristics may directly or indirectly affect their ability to obtain high-quality care and attain desired health outcomes. Lewis and colleagues[10] view vulnerable populations as being comprised of 2 distinct but overlapping populations: the clinically at-risk population and the socially disadvantaged population. The clinically at-risk populations are comprised of patients with clinical conditions or risk factors that render them at risk for poor health and medical outcomes. Tierney[11] argues that people are not born vulnerable; they are made vulnerable. She adds that different axes of inequality combine and interact to systems of oppression—systems that relate directly to differential levels of social vulnerability.

Marginality is defined as "an involuntary position and condition of an individual or group at the margins of social, political, economic, ecological, and biophysical systems, that prevent them from access to resources, assets, services, restraining freedom of choice, preventing the development of capabilities, and eventually causing extreme poverty."[12 (p3)] Utilizing the concept of disparities and equity, Baah and colleagues[13] identify terms such as social exclusion as synonymous with marginalization, ostracism, and rejection and loneliness as consequences of marginalization. Consequently, individuals who are marginalized, or socially excluded, are in a position with limited protection and have the highest risk of poor health outcomes.[13] Marginalized groups have often suffered discrimination or been excluded from society and the health-promoting resources it has to offer. Undeservingly, they have been pushed to society's margins, with inadequate access to key opportunities.[14] Marginalization is also associated with structural and social inequality, which is a result of intentional rejection with lowering to a powerless position in society that severely restricts survivability.[13] This act of rejection is continued through viewpoints such as racism, classism, ableism, and many other lethal "isms."

Even if quality care is available to marginalized and vulnerable populations, Bhatt and Priya[15] assert that there are inherent challenges that often prevent community members from being able to access healthcare or achieve their health goals. These authors add that there is an important difference between lack of presence and lack of access: services may be present in a community, but individuals may be unable or unwilling to utilize them as intended. To address this issue, Campinha-Bacote[16] developed a checklist for rendering culturally responsive care to these populations.

OPERATIONALIZING CULTURALLY RESPONSIVE SERVICES

The Six A's Checklist for Culturally Responsive Services model recommends that services to vulnerable and marginalized populations be available, accessible, affordable, acceptable, appropriate, and affirming. While many services are made available to the general public, there is limited availability of evidence-based therapies for vulnerable populations. Research has consistently demonstrated the lack of effectiveness of mainstream interventions with culturally diverse groups.[17] Moreover, although services may be available to cultural and ethnic groups, some of these programs have not been easily *accessible*. Attempts must be made to eliminate geographic, linguistic, and other barriers restricting access to services for certain populations.

Culturally responsive programs must not only be available and accessible but also must be *affordable* to culturally diverse populations. Having access to health insurance is a critical factor in reducing the current health disparities that exist among minorities and other vulnerable populations. In an attempt to reduce these disparities, the Affordable Care Act (ACA) was passed in 2010. Despite the efforts of the ACA, current data still reflect a disparity in health insurance coverage for ethnic and racial groups. For example, 9.9% of African Americans in comparison to 5.9% of European Americans were uninsured.[18]

Providing culturally *acceptable* services means that patients perceive these services to be relevant to their problem and helpful in obtaining desired outcomes. Effective patient engagement has been associated with high-quality healthcare.[19] Patients must also find healthcare services culturally *appropriate* and be willing to adopt them as their own. Failure of the patient to see services as appropriate can lead to nonadherence. Healthcare professionals must realize that nonadherence is not a patient issue but a system issue, and the problem of "Why are specific cultural groups nonadherent with programs aimed to help them?" quickly becomes restated as "What types of culturally specific services are needed to meet the health needs of specific cultural groups?"

Finally, culturally responsive services are *affirming*. Affirming services accept and validate the patient's cultural identity. Examples of services that are affirming are offering an encouraging word, identifying the patient's strengths, using positive language, making sure you know the patient's name and how they would like to be referred to, being supportive, demonstrating respect by validating the patient's concerns, and making patients feel welcomed.

CULTURAL COMPETENCE VERSUS CULTURAL HUMILITY: THE DEBATE

The changing demographics and economics of our growing multicultural world and the long-standing disparities in the health status of people from culturally diverse backgrounds have challenged healthcare professionals and organizations to consider cultural diversity as a priority. However, despite efforts to provide culturally and linguistically responsive services to our ever-growing, diverse world, healthcare organizations and healthcare professionals continue to ask the questions, "What does it mean to be a culturally competent healthcare professional or healthcare organization and how do we get there?"

Cultural competence has a history of being viewed as the cornerstone of fostering cross-cultural communication, reducing health disparities, improving access to better care, increasing health literacy, and promoting health equity.[20] However, there is an ongoing debate in the literature which maintains that a focus on developing a culturally competent healthcare workforce, though well intended, has resulted in an unintentional overemphasis on shared group characteristics and the undervaluing of unique differences of individuals. Moreover, the debate states that cultural competence fails to address the privilege and power imbalances between professionals and the clients they serve, as well as between healthcare organizations and the communities.[21]

Cultural humility is often seen as an alternative approach to that of cultural competence. Cultural humility, a term coined by Tervalon and Murray-Garcia,[22] is a dynamic and lifelong process focusing on self-reflection and personal critique. The literature reveals an inundation of articles differentiating cultural humility from cultural competence. Specifically, cultural humility (1) requires less emphasis on knowledge and competency, (2) places a greater emphasis on a lifelong commitment, (3) encourages nurturing of self-evaluation and critique, (4) addresses power imbalances, (5) promotes interpersonal sensitivity, (6) requires an attitude of openness and being egoless, (7) involves supportive interaction, 8) entails maintaining an interpersonal stance that is other-oriented, and (9) necessitates learning from differences.[16,22,23] Campinha-Bacote[16] calls for a paradigm shift in how one views cultural competence and cultural humility. This shift necessitates that cultural humility and cultural competence enter into a synergetic relationship, resulting in a combined effect that is greater than the sum of their separate effects. This synergistic relationship is embodied in the coined term, "cultural competemility."

THE PROCESS OF CULTURAL COMPETEMILITY IN THE DELIVERY OF HEALTHCARE SERVICES

The Process of Cultural Competemility in the Delivery of Healthcare Services[16] model defines cultural competemility as the synergistic process between cultural humility and cultural competence, in which cultural humility permeates each component of cultural competence: cultural awareness, cultural knowledge, cultural skill, cultural desire, and cultural encounters. The result of this permeation can be symbolically represented in a rotating ambigram. An ambigram is a word, art form, or other symbolic representation whose elements retain meaning when viewed or interpreted from a different direction, perspective, or orientation. **Fig. 1** displays an ambigram in which the word competence, when flipped or rotated spells the word humility as seen in **Fig. 2**. Thus, humility is found in competence and competence is found in humility. Each of the constructs of cultural competemility will be defined and strategies on how to allow the construct of cultural humility to permeate each component will be discussed.

Cultural awareness involves the process of conducting a self-examination and critical reflection of one's own biases toward other cultures. Cultural awareness also involves being aware of the existence of 'isms' in healthcare delivery. The 'isms' is an umbrella term to refer to a range of attitudes and behaviors that involve perceived superiority, oppression, and discrimination based on factors such as race, national origin, ethnicity, language, social class, disability, gender, sexual orientation, and identity. For example, racism is considered a fundamental cause of adverse health outcomes for racial/ethnic minorities and racial/ethnic inequities in health.[24(p105)] Koschmann and colleagues[25] call on nurses to commit to antiracism in their clinical

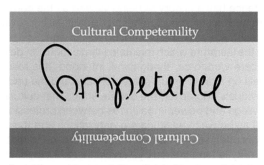

Fig. 1. Competence/humility ambigram. ©*Copyrighted by Campinha-Bacote*[16]*; not to be reprinted without permission*

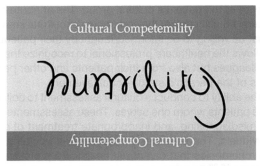

Fig. 2. Humility/competence ambigram. ©*Copyrighted by Campinha-Bacote*[16]*; not to be reprinted without permission*

practice. A commitment to antiracism should be done without shaming others. Zembylas[26] calls for "strategic empathy" as a pedagogical tool that can open up affective spaces to disrupt the emotional roots of troubled knowledge. Strategic empathy is the social and emotional skill that helps us understand the emotions, conditions, intentions, thoughts, and needs of others, in order to offer sensitive, insightful, and appropriate communication for an antiracist pedagogy. **Box 1** provides nurses with the mnemonic R.A.C.E (recognize, acknowledge, challenge, engage), as a self-examination tool that raises questions regarding one's commitment to antiracism.[16]

Healthcare professionals can allow *cultural humility* to permeate cultural awareness by intentionally and mindfully acknowledging the privilege and power inherent in their clinician role. The conscious infusion of cultural humility into the construct of cultural awareness involves the commitment of personal sacrifice. Healthcare professionals must be willing to sacrifice their prejudices and biases toward culturally different patients in order to develop cultural competemility.

Cultural knowledge is defined as the process in which the healthcare professional seeks and obtains a sound educational base about culturally diverse groups.[16] Additionally, cultural knowledge includes the integration of 3 areas: (a) health-related beliefs, practices, and cultural values of culturally and ethnically diverse populations; (b) disease incidence and prevalence among culturally and ethnically diverse populations; and (c) treatment efficacy among culturally and ethnically diverse populations.[27] The infusion of *cultural humility* into cultural knowledge allows meaningful and deliberate cultural encounters to connect with the patient as a unique, individual person,

---

Box 1
R.A.C.E: An Antiracist Pedagogy

Recognize: Do I recognize the historical, political, and social racial realities experienced daily by racial and ethnic minorities?

Acknowledge: Do I acknowledge the systematic and institutional mechanisms and power hierarchies constructed from race and race relations?

Challenge: Do I challenge and/or change aspects of a system that maintains power, privilege, and racism?

Engage: Do I engage in an understanding of the social construction, significance, and functionality of race in today's society?

Campinha-Bacote[16]

and not a stereotype of the patient's cultural group. The attribute of teachableness is necessary as cultural humility enters the component of cultural knowledge. Healthcare professionals must be willing to be informed/taught by their patients and others; for a teachable spirit allows the healthcare professional to recognize that they can learn not only from their colleagues but also from their patients and other people (cultural informants), regardless of the person's status or achievement.

Cultural skill is the ability to conduct a cultural assessment to collect relevant cultural data regarding the patients whom one serves. These assessments can prevent potential stereotyping, misdiagnosing, and inappropriate treatment of culturally and ethnically diverse individuals. The literature is saturated with cultural assessment tools, frameworks, and mnemonics that can assist healthcare professionals in conducting a cultural assessment.[16,28] To infuse *cultural humility* into cultural skill, it is suggested that healthcare professionals listen with interest and remain nonjudgmental about what they hear. Boesen[29] offers the acronym, 'ASSESS,' as a guide on how to develop consistent cultural humility: Ask questions in a humble, safe manner; Seek self-awareness; Suspend judgment; Express kindness and compassion; Support a safe and welcoming environment; and Start where the patient is at.

Cultural encounters encourage the healthcare professional to directly engage in face-to-face interactions and other types of encounters with patients from culturally diverse backgrounds to modify existing beliefs about a cultural group and prevent possible stereotyping. Continuous cultural encounters are needed to acquire cultural awareness, cultural knowledge, cultural skill, and cultural desire. Healthcare professionals must be cautious and recognize that interacting with 3 or 4 members from a specific cultural group does not make one an expert on that group. It is possible that these 3 or 4 individuals may or may not truly represent the stated beliefs, values, and practices of the specific cultural group that the healthcare professional has encountered. *Cultural humility* permeates the cultural encounter as the healthcare professional becomes mindful that every encounter is an opportunity for inquisitiveness, self-reflection, critique, and lifelong learning, and also that maintaining an open heart and mind are necessary. The Society of Hospital Medicine has developed the 5 R's of cultural humility as a self-assessment tool to help healthcare professionals cultivate cultural competemility during the cultural encounter.[30] The 5 R's include *reflection* ("What did I learn from this patient encounter?"), *respect* ("Did I treat the patient respectfully?"), *regard*, ("Did unconscious biases drive this cultural encounter?"), *relevance* ("How was cultural humility relevant in this encounter?"), and *resiliency* ("How was my personal resiliency affected by this cultural *encounter*?").

Cultural desire is the motivation of the healthcare professional to "want to" (as opposed to "have to") engage in the process of becoming culturally aware, culturally knowledgeable, culturally skillful, and also seeking cultural encounters. This form of motivation requires passion. Healthcare professionals must become anguished at the social justice issues faced by our growing culturally diverse world and the severe inequalities that exist in healthcare. We must not forget the US Surgeon General's report, "Mental Health: Culture, Race, and Ethnicity,"[31] that documented racial and ethnic disparities in mental healthcare surrounding issues of misdiagnosis, underutilization, overrepresentation, and improper treatment. Explanations are multifaceted; however, there is evidence to support that these racial and ethnic disparities are related to the lack of cultural competemility among healthcare professionals. A *cultural humility* lens of cultural desire dictates an understanding of social inequalities and how they affect individuals. When cultural humility saturates the cultural desire of healthcare professionals, there becomes a profound commitment to social justice actions and the virtue of serving others. This perspective commands the quality of seeing the greatness in others and coming into the realization of the dignity and worth of others.

As nurses begin, continue, or enhance their journey toward cultural competemility, they must address the question, *"Have I humbly 'ASKED' myself the right questions?"* The mnemonic, "ASKED," represents the self-examination questions regarding one's cultural **a**wareness, **s**kill, **k**nowledge, **e**ncounters, and **d**esire (**Box 2**). While the "ASKED" mnemonic model can assist nurses in informally assessing their level of cultural competemility, the nurse may want to conduct a more formal self-assessment. The Inventory for Assessing the Process of Cultural Competemility Among Healthcare Professionals is a formal self-assessment tool that is based on The Process of Cultural Competemility in the Delivery of Healthcare Services model.[16] This instrument can provide a more robust form of self-evaluation.

Case Presentation

Ms Mena Lima is a 74-year-old second-generation Cape Verdean woman who presents to your outpatient clinic with an elevated temperature, cough, and general aches and pains. On reviewing her medical records, you find that she has a history of hyperlipidemia and depression. You also note that she has been nonadherent in taking her medication, as well as other treatment interventions that have be prescribed to her. How would you provide care for Ms Lima utilizing using the 6 constructs found within Campinha-Bacote's model, The Process of cultural Competemility in the Delivery of Healthcare Services (ie.e., cultural humility, cultural awareness, cultural knowledge, cultural awareness, cultural desire, cultural encounter)?

STRUCTURAL COMPETENCY

There is also need for structural competency among healthcare professionals in rendering care to vulnerable and marginalized populations.[32] Whereas cultural competemility focuses on identifying clinician bias and improving healthcare professional-patient communication, structural competency emphasizes diagnostic

---

Box 2
The Process of Cultural Competemility in Health Care: Have I Humbly 'ASKED' The Right Questions?

Awareness: Am I aware of my prejudices and biases, as well as the presence of racism and other 'isms?'

Skill: Do I know how to conduct a culturally/racially specific history that includes a culturally specific physical, mental health, medication, and spiritual assessment?

Knowledge: Do I know about different cultures' worldview, disease and health conditions, health disparities/inequities, social determinants of health, and the field of biocultural ecology?

Encounters: Do I have sacred and unremitting encounters with people from cultures different than mine and am I committed to resolving cross-cultural/racial conflicts?

Desire: Do I really "want to" engage in the process of cultural competemility and address the social justice issues of inequalities and inequities that exist in healthcare?

©Copyrighted by Campinha-Bacote[16]; not to be reprinted without permission

recognition of the economic and political conditions that produce and racialize inequalities in health in the first place.[33] In the process of becoming structurally competent, healthcare professionals must be cognizant that there are structural factors that place individuals or populations (such as marginalized and vulnerable populations) at risk for negative health outcomes. Structural competency requires healthcare professionals to develop a set of skills which allows them to understand the impact of social structures and how these structures and conditions produce and racialize inequalities in health to marginalized and vulnerable populations.

Metzl and Hanson[34] identify 5 intersecting skill-sets that shape the paradigm of structural competence. First, healthcare professionals must recognize the multiple structures that shape clinical interactions. This involves recognition of how economic, physical, and sociopolitical forces impact healthcare decisions. The second skill is to develop an extraclinical language of structure to shift beyond hospitals or clinics by understanding social structures as they pertain to illness and health in community settings. It mandates attention to infrastructure structures such as social determinants of health, health disparities, or epigenetics. The third skill is the need to rearticulate cultural presentations in structural terms to acknowledge the deeper ways in which complex cultural structures produce inequalities and create barriers to inclusion. The fourth skill of structural competency calls for the acknowledgment that structures that shape health and illness are neither timeless nor immutable but rather reflect specific financial, legislative, or cultural decisions made at particular moments in time.[34] The final skill of structural competency is the trained ability to recognize the limitations of structural competency. Structural competence cannot be addressed by an individual alone.

Bourgois and colleagues[35] offer healthcare professionals the Structural Vulnerability Assessment Tool to improve understanding of how social conditions and practical logistics undermine the capacities of patients to access healthcare, adhere to treatment, and modify lifestyles successfully. This tool provides probing questions in each of the following areas: financial security (ability to pay rent, utilities, phone, and so forth), residence (stable housing), risk environment (safety needs), food access (adequate nutrition; access to healthy food), social network (friends, family, or other people to help), legal status (legal issues/problems), education (literacy and health literacy), and discrimination (experiences with discrimination). These investigators contend that operationalizing structural vulnerability in clinical practice can assist healthcare professionals to think more clearly, critically, and practically about the way social structures impact an individual's health and well-being.

Clinical Reflection Question

Structural competency builds on the process of cultural competemility. As you think of becoming a structurally competent nurse, how might the knowledge that you have learned assist you in identifying the mechanisms through which structural factors shape health outcomes?

SUMMARY

The mission of Healthy People 2030[36] is to promote, strengthen, and evaluate the Nation's efforts to improve the health and well-being of all people in order that all people can achieve their full potential for health and well-being across the lifespan. This task necessitates a full spectrum of outcomes spanning from downstream, midstream, and upstream approaches. An example of a downstream nursing intervention to help reduce health disparities is to critically address patient-nurse interactions. It is well supported in the literature that interactions reflecting implicit bias are particularly concerning in the healthcare setting because they can result in lower quality care and perpetuate health disparities.[37–39] Nurses must commit to antiracism in their clinical practice. A midstream intervention to address health inequity is making clinical nursing decisions informed by the assessment of social determinants of health. Nurses working in clinics or health systems currently not screening for social determinants of health can start by advocating for the implementation of a screening system.

Moreover, Koschmann and colleagues[25] call on nurse scientists to prioritize work that exposes inequities in care quality and health outcomes. Community-based participatory research (CBPR) can be utilized in midstream and upstream approaches in the nurse researcher's journey toward cultural competemility.[40] The principles of CBPR include promotion of "equitable engagement" throughout the research process.[41(p1615)] CBPR can be used to leverage research to promote health policy to eliminate racial and ethnic health inequities. It incorporates the "Nothing about us, without us" approach to policy formulation, implementation, and evaluation/modification to enable policy change to improve health outcomes. This dictum communicates the idea that no policy should be decided by any representative without the full and direct participation of members of the group(s) affected by that policy.

In summary, nursing must play a critical role in disrupting structural barriers and transforming an individual's quality of life and health outcomes. Nurses must be engaged in an intricate dance of meeting basic needs downstream, either directly or indirectly, through linking patients with existing resources and moving upstream to advocating for healthy public policy.[42] This requires a greater engagement of nursing in advocating for the societal and policy changes needed to create a nation in which health equity is a reality. Nationally, nursing have been consistently ranked as the most trusted profession. Our voice has credibility and we must strategically use that voice to advocate for the voiceless to bring policy makers together to support policies that improve health equity and health disparities.[43]

CLINICS CARE POINTS

- Cultural competemility includes the constructs of cultural humility, cultural awareness, cultural knowledge, cultural skill, cultural desire, and cultural encounters.

- Structural competency requires healthcare professionals to understand the impact of social structures and how these structures and conditions produce and racialize inequalities in health.

- Address health inequities by making clinical nursing decisions informed by the assessment of social determinants of health.

- Nonadherence is not a patient issue, but a system issue, and the problem of "Why are specific cultural groups non-adherent with programs aimed to help them?" must be reframed as "What types of culturally specific services are needed to meet the health needs of specific cultural groups?"

- Continuous cultural encounters are needed to acquire cultural awareness, cultural knowledge, cultural skill, and cultural desire.

- Healthcare professionals must be cognizant that there are structural factors that place individuals or populations (such as marginalized and vulnerable populations) at risk for negative health outcomes.

DISCLOSURE

I do not have any commercial or financial conflicts of interest to disclose and received no funding for this project.

REFERENCES

1. National Academies of Sciences, Engineering, and Medicine. (2021). The Future of nursing 2020–2030: Charting a path to achieve health equity. The National Academies Press.
2. American Association of Colleges of Nursing. (2021). The essentials: Core competencies for professional nursing education. https://www.aacnnursing.org/AACN-Essentials.
3. International Council of Nurses. The ICN code of ethics for nurses 2021.
4. Moss M, Phillips J. *Health equity and nursing: Achieving equity through policy*, population health, and interprofessional collaboration. NY: Springer Publishing Company, LLC; 2021.
5. American Nurses Association. Code of ethics for nurses with interpretive statements 2015.
6. Pacquiao D, Basuray Maxwell J, Ludwig-Beymer P, et al. Integration of population health, social determinants, and social justice in transcultural nursing and culturally competent care: White paper by the scholars education interest group. J Transcult Nurs 2023;1–3. Silver Spring, MD: American Nurses Association.
7. Pacquiao DF, Douglas MK. Social pathways to health vulnerability: Implications for health professionals. NY: Springer; 2019.
8. National Collaborating Centre for Determinants of Health. (2013). Let's talk: Populations of the power of language. Antigonish, NS: National Collaborating Centre for Determinants of Health. ST. Francis University.https://nccdh.ca/images/uploads/Population_EN_web2.pdf.
9. Waisel D. Vulnerable populations in healthcare. Current Opinion in Anesthesiology 2013;26(2):186–92.
10. Lewis V, Larson B, McClurg A, et al. The promise and peril of accountable care for vulnerable populations: A framework for overcoming obstacles. Health Aff 2012;31(8):1777–85.
11. Tierney K. Disasters: a sociological approach. NY: Wiley & Sons; 2019.
12. Gatzweiler F, Baumuller H, von Braun J, Ladeburger C. Marginality: Addressing the root causes of extreme poverty. ZEF working paper 77. Bonn: Center for Development Research, University of Bonn; 2011.
13. Baah B, Teitelman A, Riegel B. Marginalization: Conceptualizing patient vulnerabilities in the framework of social determinants of health – An integrative review. Nurs Inq 2019;26(1):e12268.
14. Braveman P, Kumanyika S, Fielding J, et al. Health disparities and health equity: The issue is justice. American Journal of Public Health 2011;101(S1):S149–55.
15. Bhatt J, Priya B. Ensuring access to quality health care in vulnerable communities. Acad Med 2018;93(9):1271–5.
16. Campinha-Bacote J. The process of cultural competemility in the delivery healthcare services: unremitting encounters. 6th Edition. Springboro, OH: Braughler Books LLC; 2020.
17. Yates, I., Byrne, J., Donahue, S., McCarty, L. & Mathews, A. (2020). Representation in clinical trials: A review on reaching underrepresented populations in research. Clinical Researcher, 34(7). https://acrpnet.org/2020/08/10/representation-in-clinical-trials-a-review-on-reaching-underrepresented-populations-in-research/.

18. Office of Minority Health. (2019). Profile: Black/African Americans. Washington, D.C.: U.S. Department of Mental Health and Human Resources. https://www.minorityhealth.hhs.gov/omh/browse.aspx?lvl=3&lvlid=61.

19. Hickmann E, Richter P, Schlieter H. All together now–patient engagement, patient empowerment, and associated terms in personal healthcare. BMC Health Serv Res 2022;22(1):1–11.

20. Yancu C, Farmer D. Product or process: Cultural competence or cultural humility? Palliative Medicine and Hospice Care Open Journal 2017;3(1):e1–4.

21. Campinha-Bacote J. Cultural competemility: A paradigm shift in the cultural competence vs cultural humility debate– Part I. OJIN: Online J Issues Nurs 2018;24(1).

22. Tervalon M, Murray-Garcia J. Cultural humility versus cultural competence: A critical distinction in defining physician training outcomes in multicultural education. J Health Care Poor Underserved 1998;9(2):117–25.

23. Foronda C, Baptiste D, Reinhold M, et al. Cultural humility: A concept analysis. J Transcult Nurs 2016;27(3):201–17.

24. Williams D, Lawrence J, Davis B. Racism and health: Evidence and needed research. Annu Rev Publ Health 2019;40:105–25.

25. Koschmann K, Jeffers N, Heidari O. "I can't breathe": A call for antiracist nursing practice. Nurs Outlook 2020;68(5):539–41.

26. Zembylas M. Pedagogies of strategic empathy: Navigating through the emotional complexities of anti-racism in higher education. Teach High Educ 2012;17(2):113–5.

27. Lavizzo-Mourey R. Cultural competence: Essential measurements of quality or managed care organizations. Ann Intern Med 1996;124(10):919–21.

28. Purnell L, Fenkl E. *Textbook for transcultural nursing: a population appro*ach: cultural competence concepts in nursing care. NY: Springer Publishers; 2020.

29. Boesen. L. (January 17, 2012). Creating connections through cultural humility. Available at: http://www.lisaboesen.com/creating-connections-through-cultural-humility/.

30. Ansari, A. (April 25, 2017). Battling biases with the 5Rs of cultural humility. Hospitalist. https://www.the-hospitalist.org/hospitalist/article/136529/leadership-training/battling-biases-5-rs-culturalhumility.

31. U.S. Department of Health and Human Services. (2001). Mental health: culture, race, and ethnicity - a supplement to mental health: a report of the surgeon general. Rockville, MD: U.S. Department of Health and Human Services, Substance Abuse and Mental Health Services Administration, Center for Mental Health Services, National Institutes of Health, National Institute of Mental Health.

32. Davis S, O'Brien AM. Let's talk about racism: Strategies for building structural competency in nursing. Acad Med 2020;95(12S):S58–65.

33. Downey M, Gómez A. Structural competency and reproductive health. AMA Journal of Ethics 2018;20(3):211–23.

34. Metzl J, Hansen H. Structural competency: Theorizing a new medical engagement with stigma and inequality. Social Sciences and Medicine 2014;103:126–33.

35. Bourgois P, Holmes S, Sue K, et al. Structural vulnerability: Operationalizing the concept to address health disparities in clinical care. Acad Med 2017;92(3):299–307.

36. Office of Disease Prevention and Health Promotion. Healthy people 2030. Washington, DC: U.S. Department of Health and Human Services, Office of Disease Prevention and Health Promotion; 2020.

37. Schatz AA, Chambers S, Wartman GC, et al. Advancing more equitable care through the development of a health equity report card. J Natl Compr Cancer Netw 2023;21(2):117–24.
38. Richard-Eaglin A, Muirhead L, Webb M, et al. A syndemic effect: Interrelationships between systemic racism, health disparities, and COVID- 19. Nursing2022 2022;52(1):38–43.
39. Lee A, Padilla C. Causes of health inequities. Curr Opin Anaesthesiol 2022;35(3): 278–84.
40. Fitzgerald E, Campinha-Bacote J. Cultural competemility Part II: An intersectionality approach to the process of competemility. Online J Issues Nurs 2019;24(2).
41. Cacari-Stone L, Wallerstein N, Garcia A, et al. The promise of community-based participatory research for health equity: A conceptual model for bridging evidence with policy. American Journal of Public Health 2014;104(9):116–23.
42. Falk-Rafael A, Betker C. Witnessing social injustice downstream and advocating for health equity upstream: "The trombone slide" of nursing. Adv Nurs Sci 2012; 35(2):98–112.
43. DePriest K, Alexander K, Taylor J. Addressing social determinants of health: a nursing imperative to achieve health equity during covid-19 pandemic and beyond. John Hopkins Nursing Magazine; 2020.

Perceptions to Overcoming Barriers to Prenatal Care in African American Women

Katilya S. Ware, PhD, RN[a],*, Amy S.D. Lee, DNP, ARNP, WHNP-BC[b],
Mayra Rodriguez, PhD, MPH[c], Courtney H. Williams, BSc (Psychology)[d]

KEYWORDS

- Prenatal care visits • African American women • Pregnancy-related deaths
- Centering pregnancy • Group prenatal care

KEY POINTS

- Major barriers reported to prenatal care are related to issues at the individual and provider level.
- Facilitators to prenatal care utilization include improving access, providing education, family support, and providers taking time to listen and explain conditions to their patients is essential in overcoming barriers to prenatal care.
- Establishing rapport and gaining trust are essential components to retaining African American women in health promotion activities.

Trends in pregnancy-related deaths in the United States have increased over the last 2 decades.[1] Approximately 700 women die each year in the United States from pregnancy-related complications.[2] African American (AA) women are disproportionately affected and experience higher rates of complications from pregnancy compared with other racial groups regardless of socioeconomic status, education levels, and geographic location.[1,3,4] Pregnancy-related deaths affect AA women at a rate three to four times higher than their White counterparts.[5] The underlying cause for these disparities is not fully understood but has been thought to include factors involving the patient (eg, as job constraints, financial constraints, and lack of childcare, social support, and education/health literacy), practitioner (eg, relationship and experience with health care providers), and health care system (eg, lack of health insurance and transportation).

---

[a] Auburn University College of Nursing, 710 South Donahue Drive, Auburn, AL 36849, USA;
[b] Capstone College of Nursing 3006, Box 870358, Tuscaloosa, AL 35487, USA; [c] Edward Via College of Osteopathic Medicine Auburn, 910 South Donahue Drive, Auburn, AL 36832, USA;
[d] Auburn University College of Nursing, 710 South Donahue Drive, Auburn, AL 36832, USA
* Corresponding author.
E-mail address: kwh0011@auburn.edu

Nurs Clin N Am 59 (2024) 121–129
https://doi.org/10.1016/j.cnur.2023.11.010
0029-6465/24/Published by Elsevier Inc.
nursing.theclinics.com

A pregnancy-related death occurs because of a complication or chain of events initiated or aggravated by the physiologic effects of pregnancy not accidental or intentional in nature.[3] More than 80% of pregnancy-related deaths are preventable.[6] Developing and implementing solutions aimed at reducing pregnancy-related deaths are essential.

BACKGROUND

Ideally, a woman receives prenatal care services as soon as she learns of the pregnancy. Prenatal care visits can occur as early as 6 weeks or after a woman's first missed period. The prenatal period is essential as it allows providers to gain understanding of the mother's overall health, screen for conditions that are unique or coincidental to pregnancy, and provide prompt and adequate treatment. Previous studies have found that prenatal care services are often underused or delayed until the second or third trimester in AA women. A major factor associated with lower prenatal care utilization in AA women is distrust in the health system because of historical atrocities such as the Tuskegee Syphilis Study.[1]

Because faith-based institutions are one of the most trusted places where support and resources are received in AA communities, partnerships with faith-based leaders are essential in health promotion[5,7,8]. Health promotion interventions implemented in AA churches are effective in improving health behaviors and outcomes.[9] Studies using a faith-based care model strongly support feasibility and extend reach of church-based interventions beyond the church and the communities they serve.[10] This study investigated the feasibility of a faith-based centering pregnancy model (FBCPM).

Centering pregnancy is a model of group prenatal care composed of three major components: health assessment, education, and support. This type of care model allows women to come together as a support system while receiving prenatal care and participating in education. Centering pregnancy may aid in continuity of care, including consistency of provider(s), coordinated and comprehensive services, and care that values patient opinions.[11] Although few studies have investigated the effectiveness of group prenatal care in AA women, the use of the model has been associated with increased satisfaction and improved birth outcomes.[12] There is no study to date that has examined an FBCPM for improving attendance to prenatal care visits in AA women.

An inclusive research approach was used to engage AA women, health experts, and faith-based leaders to promote adherence to prenatal care services. The purpose of this study was to investigate the barriers and facilitators impacting the utilization of prenatal care services by AA women, assess the feasibility of an FBCPM as an intervention, and explore the role of faith-based institutions in promoting maternal health, aiming to inform the development of tailored health care strategies for improved maternal health outcomes. Although previous studies have identified barriers to prenatal care in AA women, few have proposed solutions that include a faith-based approach aimed at increasing attendance to improve maternal health outcomes.

METHODS

A qualitative approach was used to conduct the study and gain an in-depth understanding of facilitators and barriers to prenatal care from the perspective of AA woman, health experts, and faith-based leaders. To gain this in-depth understanding, focus group and individual semistructure interviews were conducted. Lived experiences provide meaning to each person's perspective.[13]

Participants and Setting

A snowball sampling method was used to recruit participants. Snowball sampling is one of the most common forms of purposeful sampling that involves locating a few key participants who easily meet the criteria established for participation in a study.[14] Flyers were also used as a recruitment strategy. Participants were categorized into the following groups: AA women, health experts, and faith-based leaders. Women were eligible for participation in the study if they were AA race, female, between the age of 19 and 44 and were currently pregnant or delivered within the last 2 years. Health experts were eligible for participation in the study if they were a medical doctor, nurse practitioner, nurse, childbirth unit manage, or director and could speak English. Faith-based leaders were eligible for participation if they identified as a pastor, deacon, secretary, or preacher's wife/first lady in an AA church and could speak English. All participants resided in the southeastern United States.

Ethical Considerations

Before conducting the study, approval was obtained from the university institutional review board. Informed consent was obtained before each interview. Individuals who participated via Zoom were provided the opportunity to turn off their camera and display a pseudonym during the interview to maintain confidentiality. All electronic data files were kept strictly confidential in a secure folder, and access was restricted to members of the research team. Participant information was kept confidential in a locked file cabinet and access was restricted to the primary researcher.

Procedures

Data were collected more than 4 months (October 2021–November 2021) via semistructured individual or focus group interviews using an interview protocol. To ensure consistency, the same member of the research team functioned as the moderator during interviews. Each interview began with an introduction to the research topic. Following the introduction, consent was obtained to record the interviews using a digital recording device or virtually through use of Zoom videoconferencing software. Although an interview guide was used, probing questions were used whenever appropriate. The duration of each interview ranged from approximately 45 to 90 minutes. Interviews were conducted until data saturation was achieved. Audio recordings from interviews were imported and transcribed using NVivo Transcription qualitative analysis software. Transcriptions were compared with written and audio recorded notes to ensure trustworthiness of the data.

Measures

The Health Belief Model was used to develop interview questions specific to maternal health. Interview questions were validated by an expert on qualitative approaches to ensure questions aligned with the study aims. The guide consisted of one general introductory question specific to each participant group to promote engagement. The guide also contained five open-ended questions to allow participants the opportunity to provide in-depth responses. Two closing questions were used to conclude the interview. Sample interview questions are provided in **Table 1**.

Data Analysis

Data were analyzed using thematic analysis. Transcriptions for each interview organized into three categories: AA women, health experts, and faith-based leaders. Four researchers (KW, AL, MR, and CW) independently analyzed transcript data into codes using first and second cycle coding methods: holistic, in vivo, and versus

Table 1 Semi-structured Interview Questions	
Introductory Questions	When did you become pregnant or when did you deliver? (AA women) What is your experience with delayed care during pregnancy or continuum of care after delivery? (health experts) What is your experience with expectant mothers or new mothers in the church?
Direct Questions	What barriers (individual or social) do you see related to care during pregnancy?
	What barriers do you see during care after pregnancy, specifically during the first year after pregnancy?
	How can these barriers be improved?
	What do you think are the benefits to receiving continued care from a provider?
	How susceptible are AA women to poor maternal outcomes?
	How serious are these problems for an AA woman and her baby?
Probing Questions	Could you say something more about that?
Closing Questions	Is there anything else you would like to share?
	Are there any questions that you think I should have asked?

codes were clustered into themes to gain an in-depth understanding of facilitators and barriers to prenatal care in AA women and the feasibility of a faith-based centering pregnancy model. Member checking and peer debriefing were strategies used to enhance the quality of thematic analysis.

RESULTS

Eight AA women participated in an individual semistructured interview. Seven faith-based leaders participated in a focus group interview: three females and four males. One additional male faith-based leader participated in an individual semistructured interview. All health experts were female: six participated in individual semistructured interviews and two in a group interview.

Schedule conflicts, inadequate number of providers, access, lack of knowledge, and feeling unheard or rushed by the provider were major themes that emerged related to barriers to care during pregnancy from the perspective of AA women, health experts, and faith-based leaders. The need for education emerged as a theme among all three groups as a strategy to overcome barriers to care during pregnancy. Health experts and AA women also expressed it was necessary to improve access to overcome barriers. Family support emerged as an additional theme specific to faith-based leaders. Specific to AA women providers taking time to listen and explain during visits was also essential.

Time, incentives, and appropriate platforms for advertisement were themes that emerged specific to recruitment of AA women for health promotion activities. However, depending on the type of activity, liability was a theme that emerged among health experts. Establishing rapport and gaining trust were a critical component associated with retention of AA women for health promotion activities.

Barriers Related to Care During Pregnancy

Schedule conflicts and related to work, life, or school and inadequate number of providers were major themes that emerged from AA women and faith-based leaders. One

AA woman stated: "The doctor's office that I did go to, they would only see their prenatal patients during a certain day and at a certain time…I think they only saw us like Monday morning or Tuesday morning or something like that, and me being in school, they kind of posed a potential problem for me because I couldn't come in the mornings because I had class." A female faith-based leader had this to say: "When you're a working mother, a single mother, you don't have time to go to these doctor's appointments…and they're not willing to work with you as far as the time frame so you can get off work. I had to schedule my doctor's appointments on my lunch break, so I didn't go to lunch. I went to the doctor's office, and I would just change it up at work.…My job was flexible, but everybody don't have that convenience."

Access was another major overarching theme specific to data reported by AA women and health experts. The most reported barriers that prevented access to care were lack of insurance, transportation, and childcare. One AA woman explained: "Insurance is one thing, and then I know I know a lot of women are able to get Medicaid but some of them aren't. It seems like they make Medicaid more difficult to get these days. It seems like it is. I know a couple of people where their income is like a dollar or two too much and then they deny them of getting Medicaid. So, then that prevents the person from getting prenatal care like they need to because they have to come out of pocket with more money. Or they don't have it to come out of pocket…more money or things like that…and then transportation. They don't like to bother people for rides, and they don't have a way to supply their own ride." One health care expert had this to say: "One, I guess probably a major barrier and in many instances is transportation. So, whether it's lack of access to transportation or lack of funds in order to get here…If people don't have like a private vehicle, if they have to ask someone to bring them to the doctor, you have issues with kind of coordinating schedules for somebody to bring them or if somebody is charging them to come or if they're having to pay for gas. So that's certainly an issue. Sometimes it's work. Their schedule doesn't really allow them the opportunity to come, you know, as often as we schedule an appointment. Sometimes it's childcare because at this point, it's particularly since COVID has been an issue. We've not allowed children into the office."

The *lack of knowledge* related to the importance of prenatal care was a theme specific to health experts as a barrier to prenatal care. One health expert stated: "Um, a lot of the women, especially if they've already had a baby, they feel like they already know what's going to go on, so they don't feel the need to come and see the doctor." Another health expert had this to share: "Sometimes it's a mindset. You know, sometimes you see higher order pregnancies where this is my fourth baby. I kind of know what to do. I'll come here and there or if there's a problem." A third health expert had this to say: "I think the greatest barrier is the lack of education and everyone assumes they know that prenatal care is important and assumes that they know what prenatal care looks like. But they don't. They don't know that they're supposed to be going on once a month for the first 28 weeks, every 2 weeks at that point, and then once a week at 36 weeks. They're not told that."

Specific to AA women *feeling unheard or rushed by the provider* was a major theme that emerged. Women shared they did not feel that their questions were important based on interactions with the provider. One AA female shared this: "I felt kind of rushed, and it was like I felt like brushed off like, OK, we got to get you in and out. So, you know, and there was one thing about I was reading where you could possibly use like oils for massages help kind of like, you know, lower the percentage of tearing when you delivered. And so, when I brought it up to one of the doctors, he didn't even like go into like, I don't know, he was like since it's your first time you're still gone probably tear so whatever. So, it was like. Okay. So that discouraged me from wanting to ask questions or things that I was interested in because it was just like I felt rushed and it was just like, you know, like it wasn't important." Another AA woman shared this about her experience "She was in a rush a lot, I felt like and I really wanted to do a vaginal birth after cesarean (VBAC). But I didn't get there, to sit her down and talk to her. Like to tell her, I want you to talk to me and tell me why. Explain to me, you know like why we can't do this and what, you know, the risk and all that kind of stuff." She also shared: "People are rushing at the bedside. Yes, physicians are overwhelmed. I get it. But I think and this is just my personal opinion, people are rushing at the bedside. They're not taking that extra time to talk to their patients."

Improving Barriers to Care During Pregnancy

Education was a major theme that derived from all participant groups. Women reported not knowing the importance of attending all prenatal care visits and indicated that if were explained it would increase the likelihood for people to adhere to appointments. However, AA women expressed that the importance of *providers taking time to listen and explain* during appointments was essential in helping them feel like they are heard, and their concerns are important. One AA woman had this to say: "I think there is a lack of doctors in certain areas. There's, I think, a big shortage. And so, to find someone who really relates to, you know…I'm not in the medical field. And so, it's like just explaining certain things to you. I don't want this to be like a burden on the doctor things I should know… I didn't want to seem goofy but I wanted the doctor to actually answer my questions and say, this is what happens. This is what happens, you know? And so, I didn't really get that."

Suggestions to *improve access* were related to offering transportation, assistance with insurance, and appointment flexibility. Health experts explained some women were aware of the availability of public transportation as a resource in commuting to doctor's appointments, but sometimes barriers related to childcare prevented use of this resource. In addition, women who have used the service have reported that it is not always on time and causes them to arrive to their appointment late. One health expert had this to say: "I heard from the patients I take care of; it would just add to the problems…they would be an hour late picking me up and I didn't have anybody to watch my kids." Appointment flexibility was important as it related to work, life, and school. One AA woman stated, "So if you have a child and nobody to keep your other child, you can't bring them to the prenatal appointment. So how are you going to come to the prenatal appointment if you don't have anybody to keep your baby and if they don't work around, you know, to make it where you can come while your child is in school or while your child's in daycare? That poses a problem too."

Faith-based leaders viewed *family* support as an essential component to overcoming barriers related to prenatal care. One faith-based leader had this to say: "These girls need support, they need help because at the end of the day, they're the one's that gotta take care of their child. Nobody is going to help her, you know, but her. She's got to wake up in the middle of the night. She's got to feed it. She's got to clothe it. She's gotta buy diapers, you know, or if not, her family got to help her do it. It needs to be more family support instead of shaming these girls and making them feel like they're nothing. The girls are already going through enough."

Perceptions of Health Promotion Activities in Churches

AA women, health experts, and faith-based leaders expressed the need to increase health promotion activities in the church. A major theme that emerged was that health promotion activities in the church were *great and necessary*. One AA expressed: "I can talk to someone that's outside of family more like about my problems than I can do with family because I feel like they can better understand where I'm coming from other than what family do, because they just say that it will be all right."

Recruiting and Retaining African American Women in Health Promotion Activities

All groups suggested that *time* was an important factor to consider when planning health promotion activities tailored toward AA. One AA woman stated: "Well, if it's the weekday for working moms, it should probably after hours after school hours. But then again, that might not be best if they have other children, and they have to help with the after-school duties. So probably on the weekend, Saturday or maybe even Sundays after church and after church service." Health experts did express concerns related to *liability* with implementation of an FBCPM. In addition, all groups indicated *incentives* were essential for the purposes of recruitment and retention. One AA women expressed: "You're going to get them there by something free... Food, goodie bags, gift cards. Just free." In addition to offering incentives, faith-based leaders and AA women shared that *advertisement* was important and suggested the use of printed and electronic flyers posted on various social media platforms. Specific to retention, faith-based leaders, and AA women expressed it was critical to *establish rapport and gain trust*.

DISCUSSION

This study examined facilitators and barriers to prenatal care from the perspective of AA women, health experts, and faith-based leaders. Findings show that AA women experience major barriers to prenatal care services at the individual and provider level. Schedule conflicts, inadequate number of providers, access, lack of knowledge, and feeling unheard or rushed by the provider were emergent themes related to barriers to prenatal care. Findings related to access specific to transportation and insurance are consistent with previous research identifying accessibility as a significant barrier to prenatal care services in AA women.[15] AA participants in this study were from diverse backgrounds with various geographic locations (rural or urban), educational and income levels and still experienced similar barriers. Additional barriers to prenatal care service utilization was such as childcare, transportation, negative caregiver qualities, and a shortage of providers aligned with a study that investigated barriers and facilitators to prenatal care for inner-city women in Canada from the perspective of health experts suggesting race may not be a factor associated with the disparity.[16] However, poor-patient provider interaction among minority groups has been linked to disparities in health care.[17]

Education, providers taking time to listen and explain, improving access, and family support were themes emergent to facilitators of prenatal care services. Health experts in previous studies have suggested increasing access to resources could aid in improved utilization of prenatal care services.[16] In addition, support systems have been associated with better utilization of prenatal care services in AA women.[17]

Although trust has been strongly linked to the church in AA community, it still serves as an essential and necessary component to health promotion activities in AA communities. Previous studies have found that trusting relationships with health care providers can improve utilization of prenatal care services.[17] Therefore, the health care provider taking the time to listen and explain the status of the pregnancy to AA women is essential.

SUMMARY

This study provides health experts and researchers understand facilitators and barriers to prenatal care for AA women. The identified challenges, including schedule conflicts, limited access, and issues of trust and communication, highlight the urgency for health care providers to adapt their approaches. By acknowledging these barriers, providers can better tailor their care to the specific needs of Black women, ultimately leading to improved maternal health outcomes.

The study also highlights the importance of implementing strategies that offer flexibility in scheduling, prioritize comprehensive education, and foster patient-centered communication. Furthermore, addressing access issues, promoting community partnerships, and ensuring culturally competent care are essential steps in bridging the gap in prenatal care disparities.

Health care providers must remember that trust is at the core of effective care. Building and maintaining trust with patients should be a fundamental aspect of their practice. By creating a supportive, nonjudgmental health care environment, providers can establish a foundation on which improved maternal health outcomes can be achieved.

In the effort to enhance maternal health for AA women, findings from this study encourage providers to adapt their approaches and engage with community resources, such as faith-based institutions, to address the unique challenges faced by this population. This proactive shift toward patient-centered and culturally sensitive care has the potential to break down the barriers that have historically hindered access to prenatal care. Ultimately, by implementing these strategies, health care providers can play a vital role in improving the health and well-being of AA women and their children.

CLINICS CARE POINTS

- Patient-Centered Communication: Taking the time to actively listen to patients' concerns and providing clear explanations of their health status, treatment options, and any questions that may have, fostering trust and engagement in care.

- Flexible Scheduling: Offer flexible appointment scheduling, including after work hours and weekend appointments, to accommodate the work and life responsibilities of Black women, making it easier for them to access prenatal care.

- Comprehensive Education: Provide comprehensive prenatal care education that emphasizes the importance of regular care visits, the typical prenatal care schedule, and the potential risks associated with delayed care.

- Community Partnerships: Collaborate with local faith-based institutions and leaders to establish partnerships that can provide support, education, and health promotion activities, creating a supportive community network for Black women seeking prenatal care.

- Nonjudgmental and Culturally Competent Care: Ensure that health care providers offer nonjudgmental and culturally competent care that respects the unique experiences and needs of Black women, creating an environment where patients feel valued and understood. This can help address the issue of feeling unheard or rushed during health care interactions.

DISCLOSURE

This research was supported by the Bonnie and Leo Sanderson Excellence Award. The funding source is not involved in the study design, data collection, analysis, interpretation, writing, or decision to submit the manuscript for publication.

REFERENCES

1. Collier AY, Molina RL. Maternal Mortality in the United States: Updates on Trends, Causes, and Solutions. Neoreviews 2019;20(10):e561–74.

2. Pregnancy-related deaths in the United States, Secondary pregnancy-related deaths in the United States, 2023. Available at: https://www.cdc.gov/hearher/pregnancy-related-deaths/index.html. Accessed May 2023.
3. Crandall K. Pregnancy-related death disparities in non-Hispanic Black women. Womens Health (Lond) 2021;17. https://doi.org/10.1177/17455065211019888. 17455065211019888.
4. Amankwaa LC, Records K, Kenner C, et al. African-American mothers' persistent excessive maternal death rates. Nurs Outlook 2018;66(3):316–8.
5. Shah JS, Revere FL, Toy EC. Improving rates of early entry prenatal care in an underserved population. Matern Child Health J 2018;22:1738–42.
6. Preventing pregnancy-related deaths. Secondary preventing pregnancy-related deaths. Available at: https://www.cdc.gov/reproductivehealth/maternal-mortality/preventing-pregnancy-related-deaths.html#print, 2023. Accessed May 2023.
7. Maxwell AE, Santifer R, Chang LC, et al. Organizational readiness for wellness promotion–a survey of 100 African American church leaders in South Los Angeles. BMC Publ Health 2019;19(1):1–10.
8. Woodard N, Williams RM, Fryer CS, et al. Correlates of health promotion in a community sample of African American churches. J Community Health 2020;45(4):828–35.
9.. Brand DJ. The African American Church: A change agent for health. ABNF J 2017;28(4):109–13.
10. Berkley-Patton JY, Thompson CB, Moore E, et al. Feasibility and outcomes of an HIV testing intervention in African American churches. AIDS Behav 2019;23:76–90.
11. Gadson A, Akpovi E, Mehta PK. Exploring the social determinants of racial/ethnic disparities in prenatal care utilization and maternal outcome. Semin Perinatol 2017;41(5):308–17.
12. Byerley BM, Haas DM. A systematic overview of the literature regarding group prenatal care for high-risk pregnant women. BMC Pregnancy Childbirth 2017;17:1–9.
13. Polit DF, Beck CT. Qualitative Research Design and Approaches. Philadelphia, PA: Wolters Kluwer; 2021. p. 471–96.
14. Merriam SB, Tisdell EJ. Designing your Study and Selecting a Sample. 4th edition. San Francisco CA: Jossey-Bass; 2015. p. 73–102.
15. Mazul MC, Salm Ward TC, Ngui EM. Anatomy of Good Prenatal Care: Perspectives of Low Income African-American Women on Barriers and Facilitators to Prenatal Care. J Racial Ethn Health Disparities 2017;4(1):79–86.
16. Heaman MI, Sword W, Elliott L, et al. Barriers and facilitators related to use of prenatal care by inner-city women: perceptions of health care providers. BMC Pregnancy Childbirth 2015;15(1):2.
17. Dahlem CHY, Villarruel AM, Ronis DL. African American women and prenatal care: perceptions of patient–provider interaction. West J Nurs Res 2015;37(2):217–35.

How Can Organizations Support a Culture of Care?

Kimberley Ennis, DNP, APRN-BC[a],*,
Dewi Brown-DeVeaux, DNP, BS, RN-ONC[b]

KEYWORDS

- Nursing • Caring • Health care • Organizational culture • Culture of care • Culture

KEY POINTS

- Leaders serve as the foundation of creating an organizational culture of care.
- Core values and practices of compassion are needed to create a caring culture.
- Creating a culture of care yields benefits to patients, employees, and organizational outcomes.

INTRODUCTION/HISTORY/DEFINITIONS/BACKGROUND

In today's competitive, ever-changing health care climate, organizational culture plays a key role in success. Tye and Dent[1] described culture as "the invisible architecture of the organization." In health care, a culture of care lays the foundation for compassionate, patient-centered health care delivery.[2] Notably, patients and families consider compassion the most influential factor in outcomes.[3] However, the culture of care stretches outside medical expertise and health care professionals and expands into an environment where people feel appreciated and supported. This supports improved patient satisfaction, reduced employee burnout, and enhanced collaboration and teamwork.[2,4,5]

Health care leaders must constantly seek effective strategies to foster and support a culture of care within their institutions.[6] Establishing sustainable strategies and practices that epitomize a culture of care is a multidimensional effort.[7] It involves protecting the psychological and physical well-being of both employees and patients, nurturing professional development, fostering effective communication, promoting wellness, ensuring a secure work environment, facilitating career advancement, and advocating for diversity and equity.[5]

Successful implementation demands consistent focus, clear vision, and unwavering commitment. It also necessitates the seamless integration of these initiatives into the

[a] Department of Nursing NYU Langone Health, Site Lead for Nursing and Patient Care Services, NYU Langone Othopedic Hospital, 301 East 17th Street, New York, NY 10010, USA; [b] Department of Nursing NYU Langone Health A, 10514 Flatlands 10th Street, Brooklyn NY 11236, USA
* Corresponding author.
E-mail address: Kimberley.ennis@aya.yale.edu

Nurs Clin N Am 59 (2024) 131–139
https://doi.org/10.1016/j.cnur.2023.11.014
0029-6465/24/© 2023 Elsevier Inc. All rights reserved.

very core of the organization.[6] A true culture of care should be both palpable and visible, making a lasting impression from a patient's initial encounter to an employee's first moment in the organization.

CULTURE DEFINED

The Office of Minority Health, US Department of Health and Human Services defines culture as "integrated patterns of human behavior that include language, thoughts, communications, actions, customs, beliefs, values, and institutions of racial, ethnic, religious, or social groups."[8] Human behavior lays the groundwork for a culture of care by establishing expected behaviors in line with core values.[9,10] For health care professionals, one of the most remarkable challenges is achieving a delicate balance between kindness and professional detachment to accomplish incredibly intimate tasks.[11] At times, it is easy to overlook the demanding nature of certain professional tasks executed by health care teams daily which requires care and compassion. However, evidence has suggested that the culture of a team is created by aligning behaviors with the organization's core values.[10] Once these core values are identified, the next important step is to transform them into actionable behaviors that serve as guidelines for health care professionals. Organizational leaders are instrumental in shaping the culture of care by identifying and promoting these core values.

CORE VALUES OF CARE AND LEADERSHIP

Core values shape the behaviors and decisions of health care professionals within organizations.[12] Clearly defining and promoting these values allows health care organizations to establish expectations for care delivery and interactions with colleagues, patients, and the broader community.[13] It creates a common language and a sense of purpose that strengthens compassionate behaviors, nurtures trust, and creates a supportive environment. These fundamental standards act as a compass for the organization's actions, policies, and decision-making processes. Their consistent alignment helps shape a positive, caring work environment throughout the organization.[12]

Leaders set the organizational tone by exemplifying responsibility and accountability to foster a culture of care.[13] They serve as role models that inspire others through their own conduct and expectations. Compassionate interactions with patients not only showcase empathy but also guide ethical decision-making. To further encourage this culture of care, leaders must create accountability systems that hold individuals responsible for exhibiting values and behaviors consistent with it.[13] A leadership accountability system provides a structured framework within an organization. It holds leaders accountable for their actions and the outcomes of their decisions. This system sets clear expectations, performance metrics, and regular evaluations to measure leadership effectiveness. Opportunities and rewards are implemented to incentivize goals and foster a culture of accountability. Transparency and effective communication help ensure openness and information sharing within teams. The system also offers learning and development opportunities, thus contributing to leaders' continuous improvement. Additionally, peer accountability and feedback mechanisms create a collaborative and supportive environment. Incorporating a well-structured leadership accountability system is instrumental in aligning leadership efforts with organizational objectives, promoting a culture of responsibility, and driving sustained success.[13]

Leaders shape the organizational deoxyribonucleic acid of compassion through a heightened sense of purpose and fulfillment for all involved. Navigating the dynamic landscape of today's health care industry demands profound leadership that grapples with complexities and ever-changing challenges. Health care leaders face staffing issues, budget constraints, and the mandate for excellent patient care, often amid unpredictable global or local health crises, such as pandemics. In the aftermath of the pandemic, leaders are confronting a transformed health care paradigm, where employees reevaluate their work environments and well-being.[12] The coronavirus disease 2019 (COVID-19) pandemic has had a profound impact on nursing, influencing job loyalty, retention, turnover, productivity, and engagement. The unrelenting demands and increased workload, combined with escalated health risks, have led to higher stress levels and burnout among nurses. This situation potentially diminishes job loyalty and exacerbates turnover, particularly due to safety concerns. Moreover, the strains on health care systems have necessitated adjustments in work practices, such as increased use of personal protective equipment (PPE) and changes in patient care protocols. These changes could adversely affect staff mental health, thus negatively impacting productivity and engagement. Consequently, these workforce challenges have had significant ripple effects on patient care delivery in nursing, with implications for staffing levels, continuity of care, and the overall resilience of health care systems.[13]

To adapt to these unprecedented challenges, leaders must critically evaluate their organizations, focusing especially on how they nurture employees and patients.[12] Such introspection is essential for cultivating a culture of care, where individuals feel genuinely valued, supported, and integral to the organization. A robust culture of care can significantly affect employee turnover, retention, productivity, job satisfaction, and patient outcomes. It underscores the importance of understanding the foundational principles of care and their extensive impact on organizational performance. Leadership within health care organizations carries the solemn responsibility of safeguarding the well-being of both patients and employees at every organizational level, with the cultivation of a culture of care radiating from the highest echelons of leadership.[13] Research has consistently linked caring leadership to a more positive and productive workforce, leading to favorable organizational outcomes.

PATIENT-CENTERED CARE

Prioritizing patients' needs, well-being, and preferences throughout their health care journey helps create a patient-centered approach.[14] Health care leaders can elevate the patient experience by cultivating a culture that prioritizes effective communication, shared decision-making, and active listening. Through educating health care providers about the significance of empathy and communication, leaders ensure that patients feel heard, understood, and engaged in their own care.

Coordination and continuity of care are also crucial in enhancing the patient experience.[14] Leaders should guide health care providers and departments in facilitating seamless transitions for patients with minimal disruptions. Gathering patient feedback through surveys or advisory councils allows continuous improvement in meeting patient needs. Health care organizations signal their commitment to delivering sympathetic, personalized, and compassionate care when they consistently strive to enhance the patient experience to impact patients' lives positively.

Educating staff members on patient-centered care is crucial. This approach emphasizes the need to understand and address each patient's unique needs, preferences, and values. Comprehensive training equips health care professionals with the skills and knowledge to deliver respectful, empathetic, and responsive care tailored to patients' concerns. Staff should learn effective communication techniques, active listening skills, shared decision-making strategies, and methods for building rapport with patients.

By emphasizing the importance of patient-centered care, leaders can empower staff members to create meaningful connections with patients, engaging them as active participants in their care and ensuring their comfort, satisfaction, and overall well-being. Ultimately, training staff members on the principles of patient-centered care leads to improved patient experiences.

FOSTERING COLLABORATION AND INCLUSIVITY

Collaboration and integrated care among health care professionals, departments, and teams are essential for patient-centered care. Leaders can promote a collaborative environment by creating platforms and spaces for knowledge exchange and best practices while promoting a culture of mutual respect and appreciation for diverse perspectives. Prioritizing inclusivity and embracing diversity in all its forms are paramount for ensuring that every staff member feels valued, respected, and included.[15] Initiatives such as diversity and inclusion training, promoting equal opportunities for career advancement, and recognizing and celebrating the contributions of individuals from different backgrounds can help foster a sense of belonging.[16]

Health care organizations can leverage their workforce's collective expertise and creativity to improve patient outcomes and increase staff satisfaction. Leaders who actively participate in regular forums and town hall meetings that highlight diverse voices provide platforms for sharing insights, suggestions, and concerns. Individuals from various disciplines and organizational levels possess a wealth of knowledge that can foster a sense of ownership and empower staff to contribute to the culture of care.

COMMUNICATION

Communication is fundamental to the daily operations and success of organizations but often presents significant challenges. Creating a culture of positive, transparent, and honest communication is essential in health care organizations.[17] Positive and effective communication is evident in interactions with patients, families, and employees. The Institute of Medicine (IOM)[18] has recognized that patient-centered care, which embodies both effective communication and technical skills, is necessary to achieve safety and quality in health care.

Fostering a culture of open communication and encouraging teamwork and collaboration allow staff members to contribute their ideas and feedback.[19] This engagement leads to improved morale, efficiency, satisfaction, and quality outcomes.[17,20] Effective communication keeps both patients and employees in health care organizations informed and aware. Intentional, frequent, thoughtful, and empathetic communication can be achieved through various channels.[17] These channels can include technological advancements like electronic medical records, meetings, emails, employee feedback platforms, text messages, communication apps, leadership town halls, patient and employee rounding, as well as organizational bulletins and newsletters.

Effective communication is significant in building a culture of care within health care organizations. Ensuring frequent, effective communication through diverse methods is essential. A culture rich in excellent communication yields many positive outcomes for both patients and employees.

PROFESSIONAL DEVELOPMENT

The professional development of nurses is essential for enhancing nursing practice and patient care delivery, especially in the context of rapidly evolving health care practices.[21] With constant updates in treatments, interventions, modalities, and care delivery models, organizations must prioritize nurses' professional development to improve care and advance practice. A LinkedIn study found that 94% of workers are more likely to stay with an organization that invests in their learning and career growth.[22] Therefore, it is necessary to understand the factors that influence professional development.

Continuing professional development not only sustains competence but also introduces new skills and creates a space for career advancement.[23] By offering opportunities for professional development, organizations improve patient care outcomes and enhance employee retention, engagement, and satisfaction.[21] When organizations invest in their employees' professional development, it demonstrates a commitment to employee learning and growth. Providing these opportunities empowers nurses, expands their knowledge, improves their practice, and positively impacts patient outcomes. It also boosts their confidence and opens doors for career advancement.[21]

MENTORSHIP

The implementation of mentorship programs in health care organizations benefits not only nurses and health care employees but also the organizations themselves. These programs cultivate a culture of care and offer essential support, learning opportunities, and avenues for growth and development. Mentorship bridges novice and experienced nurses, thus fostering relationships that instill a deep sense of belonging.[24]

Mentorship programs are tailored to the specific needs of employees and offer a range of lasting advantages, including heightened job satisfaction, improved retention rates, and increased engagement among staff.[24] Formal mentorship programs can be either formal, featuring structured objectives and assigned mentor-mentee pairs, or informal, allowing for more flexible, self-selected mentor-mentee relationships with less-defined goals. By providing a supportive environment, mentorship helps dispel longstanding negative perceptions, such as the perception of "nurses eating their young," thus contributing to a more caring and engaged workforce within the organization.

ENGAGEMENT AND WELLBEING

Promoting employee engagement and well-being leads to improved patient care and outcomes, as employees are more likely to provide compassionate care when they feel valued, supported, and engaged.[25] Health care leaders can prioritize employee well-being by implementing policies and practices that encourage work-life balance and a supportive work environment.[26] A culture of open communication and teamwork allows staff members to contribute their ideas and feedback, thus enriching the work environment.[19] Forward-looking organizations understand the importance of considering the totality of the workplace environment and centering employees in policy and practice redesign.[19]

Investment in employee engagement and well-being not only fosters a positive work environment but also augments staff morale, reduces burnout, and ultimately improves patient experiences and outcomes. Health care providers face daily stressors, including long hours, exposure to infectious diseases, ethical dilemmas, work-related violence, and demanding physical and emotional labor, often exacerbated by insufficient staffing.[27] The COVID-19 pandemic has further exacerbated these challenges, spotlighting the urgent need for wellness-focused health care systems.[26] Unaddressed stressors can significantly impair patient care delivery.[28] Organizations must, therefore, foster a culture that actively supports the physical and psychological health of health care professionals. In this era, prioritizing wellness has never been more crucial; it serves as the foundation for vigilant monitoring, empathetic patient care, and unwavering advocacy.[28]

Many stressors in nursing work environments can lead to diseases and injuries, emphasizing the importance of proactive wellness initiatives.[27] Effective measures include establishing respite rooms, wellness spaces, and resource carts, as well as distributing stress relief kits and conducting wellness rounds led by leadership.[29] Additionally, forming community wellness partnerships, offering mindfulness training, and providing childcare resources are essential for supporting the health and well-being of nurses.[26] Equally significant are mental health resources, work-life balance promotion, stress-reduction strategies, coping mechanisms, and nutritional guidance.[26] Organizations can further enhance well-being by encouraging practices such as meditation, nurturing personal connections, spending time with pets, journaling, participating in yoga, and practicing mindfulness. These tools alleviate stress and cultivate a culture centered on care and well-being.[26]

SAFETY

Creating a safe environment for both receiving and providing health care is essential. Establishing an organizational culture that prioritizes the safety of patients and staff signifies a caring approach.[30,31] Notably, health care settings are among the most hazardous occupational environments, with nurses often exposed to various health risks.[32] In fact, injuries and illnesses among health care workers occur at almost twice the national average. While patient safety is essential, the well-being of health care workers and nurses is equally important. Thus, an organization's commitment to a safe work environment is a foundational element of a caring culture.

Concern for nurses' safety manifests in how an organization safeguards them from workplace violence, injuries, and multiple environmental hazards: biological, chemical, physical, ergonomic, and psychological.[30,31] The pandemic has further highlighted the importance of adequate PPE. Cultivating a culture of care starts with safety and having protocols and policies that are frequently reviewed and aligned with national and local safety guidelines. Effective safety management also involves a reliable incident reporting system for escalating potential or actual safety issues, as well as procedures for analyzing and addressing reported safety concerns.

Maintaining adequate training, education, and awareness of resources and equipment is essential for providing safe care.[30,31] This requires regular evaluations and improvements in safety measures. Adequate staffing is also integral to creating a safe and caring work environment as it prevents workplace injuries and boosts performance and efficiency. According to the American Nurses Association, adequate staffing contributes to "improved patient outcomes and greater satisfaction for both patients and staff." The International Council of Nurses asserts that every nurse has the right to work in an environment that is free from the risk of injury or illness.[33]

Organizations should consider all aspects that influence a safe environment. Occupational injuries and illnesses can lead to psychological distress and job dissatisfaction, often resulting in increased staff turnover. This aggravates the existing challenges in the nursing workforce.[32] Therefore, all employees must actively participate in detecting and reporting safety concerns. Resources should be allocated for assessing and analyzing safety issues both before and after they occur. The IOM's report, "To Err Is Human," calls attention to the need to create a culture of safety in all health care organizations with substantial commitment.[18]

RECOGNITION

Nursing and health care delivery are among the most rewarding yet challenging professions. Nurses and health care providers take immense pride in delivering quality care to patients and their families, often going above and beyond the call of duty. Therefore, organizations should implement sustainable, meaningful recognition programs highlighting stories of compassion, exceptional care, and gratitude.[34,35] There is no greater appreciation than recognition from patients, families, or colleagues; such acknowledgments are both meaningful and impactful. An example of these recognition programs is the national DAISY Award, which celebrates and recognizes nurses for their extraordinary care, compassion, and kindness.

Creating recognition programs is one of the most effective methods for health care organizations to demonstrate their appreciation and care for employees. These programs improve employee engagement, recognition, and retention, and they inspire others to excel in their roles.[34,35] Meaningful recognition helps reduce burnout and increase compassion satisfaction as it mitigates compassion fatigue.[34,35] Recognition programs also enable organizations to learn more about their employees. Recognition can be expressed daily, weekly, monthly, or annually, and in various forms such as team huddles, notes, thank-you emails, or prizes. Ways to acknowledge employees' efforts include implementing programs such as employee of the month or year, national recognition awards, or creating organization-specific awards. Creating an employee recognition system is vital in building a culture of compassion, especially in a high-stress health care environment.

SUMMARY

Culture of care is critical in various contexts, particularly in health care organizations, because it fosters an environment where individuals feel respected, valued, and supported. This culture should embody well-being, teamwork, and trust. In health care organizations, creating a culture of care results in better patient experiences and clinical outcomes, and decreased burnout among staff. It is also fundamental for ethical conduct and patient-centeredness.

Overall, it underpins the essence of compassion and kindness, which forms the bedrock of the health care industry. However, creating a culture of compassion, although essential, can be challenging. It is the cornerstone of success in health care. Developing this culture starts with a comprehensive understanding of core principles, including patient-centered care, leadership, physical and psychological well-being, safety, communication, inclusivity, and professional growth.

The culture of care influences various outcomes for patients, families, nurses, and other health care employees. To foster this culture, organizations need to understand the various dynamics and scope from both patient and employee perspectives. Importantly, this responsibility falls upon organizational leadership, which must support, create, communicate, and model a culture of compassionate care. Providing compassionate care is mandatory and not a choice. With new changes in the dynamics of health care delivery, finances, and the emerging workforce, having a strong culture of care is more crucial than ever. Therefore, the commitment to compassionate care should extend beyond mere aspirations; it must become an intentional and integral part of organizational practices.

CLINICS CARE POINTS

- Implement and support structured mentorship programs within the health care organization.

- Establish interdisciplinary huddles or briefings, where team members from diverse disciplines come together to discuss patient care plans, share important updates, and address any communication barriers.
- Incorporate frequent wellness checks and provide access to resources that support mental and emotional well-being.

DISCLOSURE

I, K. Ennis, declare that I have no commercial or financial conflicts of interest and any funding sources relevant to the information described in this article. I, D. Brown-DeVeaux, declare that I have no commercial or financial conflicts of interest and any funding sources relevant to the information described in this article.

REFERENCES

1. Tye J, Dent B. Building a culture of ownership in healthcare: the invisible architecture of core values, attitude, and self-empowerment. Sigma Theta Tau International; 2017.
2. Frampton SB, Guastello S, Lepore M. Compassion as the foundation of patient-centered care: the importance of compassion in action. J Comp Eff Res 2013; 2(5):443–55.
3. Lown BA, Rosen J, Marttila J. An agenda for improving compassionate care: a survey shows about half of patients say such care is missing. Health Aff 2011; 30(9):1772–8.
4. Lee H-F, Kuo C-C, Chien T-W, et al. A meta-analysis of the effects of coping strategies on reducing nurse burnout. Appl Nurs Res 2016;31:100–10.
5. Arjaliès D-L, Funari S, Grandazi A, et al. Three propositions to help to cultivate a culture of care and broad-mindedness in academic publishing. LSE Academic Publishing; 2018.
6. Colebrooke L, Leyshon C, Leyshon M, et al. 'We're on the edge': cultures of care and universal credit. Soc Cult Geogr 2023;24(1):86–103.
7. Greenhough B, Davies G, Bowlby S. Why 'cultures of care'. Soc Cult Geogr 2023; 24(1):1–10.
8. US Department of Health and Human Services. Assuring cultural competence in health care: recommendations for national standards and an outcomes-focused research agenda. Available at: http://www.omhrc.gov/clas/. Accessed August 30, 2023.
9. Birch J, Heyes C. The cultural evolution of cultural evolution. Philos Trans R Soc Lond B Biol Sci 2021;376(1828):20200051.
10. Heyes C. Culture. Curr Biol 2020;30(20):R1246–50.
11. Campling P. Reforming the culture of healthcare: the case for intelligent kindness. BJPsych Bull 2015;39(1):1–5.
12. Odero A, Pongy M, Chauvel L, et al. Core values that influence the patient-healthcare professional power dynamic: steering interaction towards partnership. Int J Environ Res Public Health 2020;17(22). https://doi.org/10.3390/ijerph17228458.
13. Denier Y, Dhaene L, Gastmans C. 'You can give them wings to fly': a qualitative study on values-based leadership in health care. BMC Med Ethics 2019;20(1):35.
14. Fix GM, VanDeusen Lukas C, Bolton RE, et al. Patient-centred care is a way of doing things: how healthcare employees conceptualize patient-centred care. Health Expect 2018;21(1):300–7.

15. Hines-Martin V, Starks S, Hermann C, et al. Understanding culture in context: an important next step for patient emotional well-being and nursing. Nurs Clin North Am 2019;54(4):609–23.

16. Brown-DeVeaux D, Richards B. Metric-driven initiative for promoting staff diversity: plan, do, check, and act can serve as a framework. American Nurse Journal 2022;17(1):18–21.

17. Hicks JM. Leader communication styles and organizational health. Health Care Manag 2011;30(1):86–91.

18. Institute of Medicine. Preventing medication errors. The National Academies Press; 2007.

19. Wieneke KC, Egginton JS, Jenkins SM, et al. Well-being champion impact on employee engagement, staff satisfaction, and employee well-being. Mayo Clin Proc Innov Qual Outcomes 2019;3(2):106–15.

20. Men LR. Strategic internal communication. Manag Commun Q 2014;28(2):264–84.

21. Vázquez-Calatayud M, Errasti-Ibarrondo B, Choperena A. Nurses' continuing professional development: a systematic literature review. Nurse Educ Pract 2021;50:102963.

22. LinkedIn. 2018 workplace learning report. Available at: https://learning.linkedin.com/resources/workplace-learning-report-2018?src=li-scin&veh=7010d000001BicLAASv2&cid=7010d000001BicLAAS&bf=1. Accessed September 17, 2023.

23. Ross K, Barr J, Stevens J. Mandatory continuing professional development requirements: what does this mean for Australian nurses. BMC Nurs 2013;12:9.

24. Brown-DeVeaux D, Jean-Louis K, Glassman K, et al. Using a mentorship approach to address the underrepresentation of ethnic minorities in senior nursing leadership. J Nurs Adm 2021;51(3):149–55.

25. Scott G, Hogden A, Taylor R, et al. Exploring the impact of employee engagement and patient safety. Int J Qual Health Care 2022;34(3). https://doi.org/10.1093/intqhc/mzac059.

26. Pronk N, Kleinman DV, Goekler SF, et al. Promoting health and well-being in healthy people 2030. J Public Health Manag Pract 2021;27(Suppl 6):S242–8.

27. Luo M, Ding D, Bauman A, et al. Social engagement pattern, health behaviors and subjective well-being of older adults: an international perspective using WHO-SAGE survey data. BMC Publ Health 2020;20(1):99.

28. De-la-Calle-Durán M-C, Rodríguez-Sánchez J-L. Employee engagement and wellbeing in times of COVID-19: a proposal of the 5cs model. Int J Environ Res Public Health 2021;18(10). https://doi.org/10.3390/ijerph18105470.

29. Phillips TB, Wells NM, Brown AH, et al. Nature and well-being: the association of nature engagement and well-being during the SARS-CoV-2 pandemic. People and Nature 2023;5(2):607–20.

30. Wei H, Sewell KA, Woody G, et al. The state of the science of nurse work environments in the United States: a systematic review. Int J Nurs Sci 2018;5(3):287–300.

31. Hall LM. Quality work environments for nurse and patient safety. Jones & Bartlett Learning; 2005.

32. International Council of Nurses. International hospital federation, international pharmaceutical federation, world confederation for physical therapy, world dental federation, world medical association. Fact sheet: positive practice environment for health care professionals. World Health Professions Alliance; 2008.

33. International Council of Nurses. Occupational health and safety for nurses. 2023.

34. Tessema MT, Ready KJ, Embaye AB. The effects of employee recognition, pay, and benefits on job satisfaction: cross country evidence. J Bus Econ 2013;4(1):1–12.

35. O'Hara K, Correggio T, Llerena S, et al. Fostering a culture of recognition in the PACU. J PeriAnesthesia Nurs 2023;38(4):e23.

Second-Victim Phenomenon

Luci New, DNP, CRNA*, Tinisha Lambeth, DNP, NNP-BC

KEYWORDS

- Adverse events • Second-victim phenomenon • Peer support

KEY POINTS

- All health care workers regardless of background, education, training, or personal characteristics have the potential to be impacted as a second victim following adverse events.
- There are commonalities of a second victim including physical, psychological, and/or professional/social manifestations.
- Second victims follow a trajectory of stages as they progress to recovery from the event; although, for some, this might include relocation to a different practice setting or leaving the profession.
- Second victims desire a myriad of resources to meet their emotional needs following the adverse event, but the most preferred method is the support of a respected peer colleague.

INTRODUCTION

According to the World Health Organization (WHO), 1 out of 10 patients in developed countries suffer harm while hospitalized; 50% of that group are from preventable adverse events (AEs).[1] Globally, the percentage increases to 80%.[1] Following such encounters, health care workers (HCWs), henceforth referring to all levels of health care employees, manifest predictable signs and symptoms as they seek to work through the emotional trauma experienced. This is often referred to as the second-victim phenomenon (SVP).[2] This nomenclature was created by Dr Albert Wu[3] after witnessing a colleague's reactions to a medical error. He recognized the patient as the first victim in the event, but also noted the provider as the second victim (SV) who suffered as well.[3] Despite controversy over the term SV and the potential minimization of the patient's experience, this term remains in use.[4] Scott and colleagues[2] define it as follows: Second victims are health care providers who are involved in an unanticipated adverse patient event, in a medical error and/or a patient-related injury, and become victimized in the sense that the provider is traumatized by the event. Frequently, these individuals feel personally responsible for the patient outcome. Many feel as though

Department of Academic Nursing, Wake Forest University, School of Medicine, 525 Vine Street, Suite 230, Winston-Salem, NC 27101, USA
* Corresponding author.
E-mail address: lunew@wakehealth.edu

Nurs Clin N Am 59 (2024) 141–152
https://doi.org/10.1016/j.cnur.2023.11.011
0029-6465/24/© 2023 Elsevier Inc. All rights reserved.

nursing.theclinics.com

they have failed the patient, second-guessing their clinical skills and knowledge base.[2(p326)]

INCIDENCE

All in health care, regardless of job title, position, educational level, or professional level, have the potential to suffer as SVs.[2,5,6] Oftentimes, when there is an unanticipated AE, one is not in isolation as the SV; multiple team members can also be identified and affected.[6,7] The SVP is unfortunately an experience that can occur frequently following unexpected events; Huang and colleagues[8] reported approximately 70% of nurses had experienced at least 1 AE over the course of their careers, 35.8% during the prior 6 months. The AEs were graded as death related (1.1%), moderate (9.4%), mild (52.3%), and near misses (37.2%).[8] Likewise, in the Betsy Lehman report, 46% of respondents had been involved in an event the prior 12 months, and of that group, 77% had 2 or more in that timeframe, with 38% having experienced 4 or more.[6]

This phenomenon is not limited to North America as global studies also highlight and bring recognition to the emotional distress experienced following AEs.[7-17] In addition to self-identification of second victimization, colleagues who witnessed an event where there was no direct involvement suffered as well.[.5,9,10] One international study on second-victim responses to patients' suicidal events showed only 14% were directly involved in patient care at the time of the event, while 86% had an indirect role.[10]

MANIFESTATIONS OF SECOND-VICTIM PHENOMENON

Manifestations of SVP are diverse and individualized (**Table 1**). The list is not all-inclusive as symptoms can be individual to each HCW, although commonalities exist. There is no identified timeline for the reduction or disappearance of manifestations. Some either linger,[6,11,12,12] or the provider may be triggered by a similar patient or situation and experience similar symptoms as after the original event, even years later.[2,12]

One study reported nurses who cared for patients who attempted or completed suicide shared a "sense of being alone."[10(p3294)] At the time of the incident, nurses felt

Table 1
Manifestations of second-victim phenomenon

Type	Manifestation
Physical	Insomnia,[2,6,12-16] fatigue,[2,13] muscle tension,[2,6] increased heart rate,[2,6] hypertension,[2,13] rapid breathing,[2,6] indigestion,[6] nausea,[16] decreased appetite,[16] exhausted,[13,16] headaches[13]
Psychological	Sad,[2,6,15,17] depression,[2,10,13] anxiety,[2,6,13] guilt,[2,6,10,15,17] grief,[2] frustration,[2,6] shock/disbelief,[12] remorse,[2,16] scared,[14] fear,[2,6,15-17] anger,[2,6,12] doubt/loss of confidence,[2,6,15] confusion and blame,[17] low self-esteem and disheartened,[15] loneliness,[10,12,17] triggering events[2,12] repetitive/intrusive thoughts or memories,[2,12,15,17] difficulty concentrating,[2] flashbacks/reliving the event,[2,6,10] embarrassed, miserable,[16] despair,[12] ashamed,[12] hopelessness[12]
Professional/Social	Self-doubt and avoidance of patient care,[2] social discrimination,[15] second-guess career,[2] judged,[6] rejection,[17] worry about the future,[15] black-marked,[15] decreased joy/meaning in work,[6,18] worry/fear of damage to reputation[2,6]

patient care was solely their responsibility and they were responsible for saving the patient.[10] According to another study, HCWs who had to continue working without recognition of the psychological impact of the AE experienced feelings of loneliness.[17] These can become greater and persist for extended periods if coping must be done individually without support.[10] See **Fig. 1** for symptoms that have lingering effects.

HIGH-RISK SCENARIOS

Workplace violence is described as threats or acts of physical violence, harassment, intimidation, or other threatening disruptive behaviors occurring in the workplace and can range from verbal abuse to physical assaults and even homicide.[19] Psychological violence is more common than physical, with both types contributing to second-victim symptomology.[14,20,21] One study also noted an impact on social functioning in addition to the psychological and physical impact.[21] Al-Qadi[20(p7)] has proposed an operational definition of workplace violence: Workplace violence is any act or threat of physical violence (beating, slapping, stabbing, shooting, pinching, pushing, smashing, throwing objects, preventing individuals from leaving the room, pulling, spitting, biting or scratching, striking, or kicking; including sexual assault), harassment (unwanted behavior that affects the dignity of an individual), intimidation, or other threatening disruptive behavior that occurs at the worksite with the intention of abusing or injuring the target. It ranges from threats and verbal abuse (swearing, shouting, rumors, threatening behavior, nonserious threats, or sexual intimidation) to physical assaults and even homicide that creates an explicit or implicit risk to the health, well-being, and safety of an individual, multiple individuals, or property.

Society has globally emerged from the coronavirus disease 2019 (COVID-19) pandemic. As restrictions, policies, procedures, and mandates have softened, there must be consideration for the ongoing emotional distress endured by those in health care. Nurses endured manifestations of second victimization, including acute traumatic stress, anxiety, inadequate sleep, workplace violence episodes, mental health

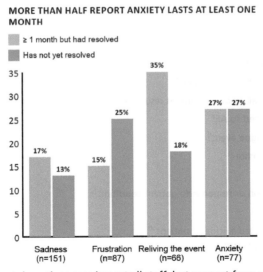

MORE THAN HALF REPORT ANXIETY LASTS AT LEAST ONE MONTH

≥ 1 month but had resolved
Has not yet resolved

Fig. 1. Difficult events in patient care impact all staff, but support from peers can help, May 27, 2021. (*Reprinted with permission from* the Betsy Lehman Center for Patient Safety. Retrieved from https://betsylehmancenterma.gov/.)

concerns, and posttraumatic stress disorder.[22] Nurses experienced overwhelming numbers of patients suffering and dying alone without the presence of family or loved ones.[22] Other frontline workers were not immune to similar symptoms, either. During the spring of 2022, the Mental Health America report[23] surveyed almost 5000 HCWs serving in allied capacities; 75% reported insomnia, physical symptoms (headaches, gastrointestinal distress, change in appetite), and 33% experienced racing and upsetting thoughts. See **Box 1** for additional high-risk scenarios.

SECOND-VICTIM OUTCOMES

One of the earliest recovery trajectories of SVs was described in 2009.[2] Since that time, other research studies have identified themes (**Table 2**) that overlap and share commonalities with prior work.

The term "burnout" was first introduced in 1974 by Dr Herbert Freudenberger and is now frequently used across all societal norms and professions to describe the impact of stress in helping professions.[25] According to the WHO, burnout is classified in the 11th Revision of the International Classification of Diseases as a syndrome resulting from unmanaged, prolonged occupational stress; however, this term does not apply to other life experiences.[26] There can exist overlapping symptoms of depression and burnout; it is vital to determine if one's experience is related to burnout or a mental health condition.[25]

Tawfik and colleagues[27] reported in their study that 77.6% of physicians involved in a major medical error event had a greater likelihood of burnout symptomology. For those experiencing burnout and involved in a medical error, there exists a potential risk of traversing the pathway of an SV. In fact, does burnout supersede errors, or

---

Box 1
High-risk scenarios for second victims

High-risk Scenarios

Medical error[6,12]

Patient death[6]

Pediatric patients[24]

Connection to patient[2,24]

Length of professional relationship[24]

Unexpected survival following patient resuscitation[12]

Patient death related to AE[8]

Unexpected colleague event[6]

Challenging interaction[6]

Near miss[8]

Delay in recognition or response to patient condition[12]

AEs[6,8]

Attempt or completed suicide of patient[10]

Workplace violence[13,14,21]

COVID-19[22,23]

Others: bomb threat, code blue[12]

Table 2
Recovery stages/themes of the second victim

Recovery Stages/Themes	Description
Chaos/Event response[2] Rescuing patients[11] Initial emotional and physical response[12]	Event recognition,[2,11,12] chaos,[2] focus on patient care and determine cause,[2,11] HCP distracted,[2] "autopilot mode,"[12(p2965)] prevent further patient consequences,[11] lacking available resources.[11]
Intrusive reflections[2] Responding psychologically after the event[15]	Self-isolation,[2] doubt,[2,15] "what if,"[2(p327),15(p168)] replay event internally,[2,15] loss of confidence.[15]
Restoring personal integrity[2] Feeling others' prejudice[15]	Seeking support from friend, colleague, family,[2] dubiety about career trajectory,[2] managing workplace gossip,[2,15] personal reflections on thoughts of colleagues[2,11] and potential lack of trust,[2] perceptions of "social discrimination" and "blackballed" by colleagues.[15(167)]
Enduring the inquisition[2] Effects on nurses[11] Professional responsibility[11] Having intrusive thoughts[15]	Ponders job security,[2,11,15] professional licensure,[2,11] legal repercussions,[2,11,15] worry,[15] fear of repeating mistake,[15] event disclosure to family,[2] physical[2] and psychosocial manifestations,[2,11] concern for others involved and empathy for colleagues.[11]
Obtaining emotional first aid[2] Needs of nurses involved in AE[11] Coping to recover after the event[15]	Seek emotional support from,[2,11] self-help strategies.[15]
Moving on[2] Drawing valuable lessons from the event[15] Taking responsibility for mistakes[15] Finding self-identity[15]	Thriving: Advocate for other professionals to minimize repeat occurrences.[2,15] Does not define professional practice on 1 event,[2] share experience with others.[15] Surviving: unable to forget event and forgive themselves.[2] Dropping out: transfer to another clinical setting,[2] leave the profession,[2,] personal sources of support, self-aacountability and organization-accountability toward AE.[15]

Abbreviations: AE, adverse event; HCP, healthcare professional.

are they contributing factors to burnout due to occupational forces? One international study found bullying acts toward nurses contributed to burnout.[13]

SVP has the potential to impact HCW staffing. The current and future projections of nursing shortages appear bleak for health care. According to the American Association of Colleges of Nursing, projections of over 200,000 openings for nurses each year will occur through 2031 (accounting for retirement and those leaving the workforce).[28] In 2022, 29% of nurses of all license types considered leaving the profession compared to 11% in 2020.[29] Diverse factors contributing to this shortage are multifactorial and beyond the scope of this article. However, when an HCW is experiencing second-victim distress, some profess to absenteeism and leaving the profession.[8,10,13,14,16,20,30]

Amit and colleagues[10] reported a positive correlation between distress experienced by the SV, a greater sense of being alone and absenteeism and turnover. In a study by Sachdeva,[14] only 6% of HCWs were absent following a workplace violence episode, whereas Lang[13] reported 22% of HCWs used sick time as a coping mechanism following reporting someone for workplace violence. Other outcomes of workplace violence have been described as well: resigning or moving positions in the organization, relocating to find another job, reducing work hours, or choosing to no longer work in their chosen profession.[13]

Similar to turnover, Scott and colleagues[2] described "dropping out"[2(p330)] as either changing, leaving the profession, or working in a different setting. It is postulated that perhaps ongoing intrusive thoughts about the event result in questioning the career path and electively leaving.[2] This decision is not necessarily viewed as a negative, as a fresh start can potentially promote healing for the SV.[2] The Betsy Lehman report identified practicing in a different clinical setting or changing careers as 2 of several coping strategies following difficult events.[6]

Rodriquez and Scott[18] evaluated a diverse group of professional levels of providers who elected to change career paths following involvement in an AE, where 64.9% failed to receive support afterward or fell short of meeting their emotional needs. An emotional labor was also described in which "clinicians regulated their emotions to be consistent with organizational expectations to suppress their emotional response to what had occurred."[18(p142)] 37% of respondents were told to remain quiet about the AE; 18% changed positions to a nonclinical role, while 17% transferred to a different department or unit.[18] Although the risk of AEs can occur anywhere in a health care setting, 36% reported less risk in their new position with 6% being outside of health care.[18]

Despite persistence and a desire to move on and "get back on the horse," some might endure challenges when attempting to do so and consider leaving the profession.[12(p2966)] Health care organizations must provide as many horses as necessary in the form of intentional support to retain staff. Organizational support can reduce second-victim distress, absenteeism, and turnover intentions, thereby allowing providers to successfully get back on the horse and remain in the saddle as long as desired.[30]

When faced with stressful events in the workforce, an HCW turns to strategies to cope, attempting to mitigate physical and psychological forces affecting them.[6,12] A resilient personality and positive outlook can prove helpful,[12] as well as prior experience with past exposures to trauma,[22] and taking time away from work.[12] Other adaptive methods include exercise,[6,12] proper diet,[12] yoga,[6] meditation,[6,12] or talking to someone.[6,12]

Individuals lacking the ability to engage in healthy coping skills may turn to maladaptive coping including substance use,[6,23] smoking more cigarettes,[13,23] and alcohol misuse.[12,13,22,23] There exists variability among research on substance use following second victimization. The Betsy Lehman report survey yielded 5% turned to substances following difficult events.[6] The Mental Health America survey reported approximately 25% of those HCWs were likely to increase substance use, including smoking, drinking, or use of substances (not defined) after 2 years into the COVID-19 pandemic,[23] and Lang reported 32% drinking more alcohol and 7% increasing cigarette smoking.[13]

Likewise, HCWs struggle to find satisfaction, joy, and meaning in their jobs as SVs. In 2007, the Institute of Health care Improvement, proposed an initiative to improve health care organizations' performance by focusing on 3 areas: (1) improving patient experience, (2) improving population health, and (3) health care cost reduction.[31] Almost a decade later, an additional aim was added to the 3; without an engaged and productive workforce, it is impossible to meet the triple aims.[32] The Quadruple Aim addresses this dilemma by creating workforce conditions that align with joy and purpose in work, ultimately resulting in an improved care experience.[32] Following AE, some HCWs report minimal work impact, while others express this loss moving forward in their career.[6,18] The Betsy Lehman survey respondents reported that 36% of those in clinical roles and 44% in nonclinical roles were not affected, while 33% and 28% (respectively) reported loss of joy.[6] Rodriquez and Scott[18] distributed a survey on joy and meaning in work both pre-event and post-event; 34% reported decreases in this area. Furthermore, over 50% experienced distress related to workplace violence, with a statistically significant association to younger, less experienced, and lower professional status HCWs.[14]

Finally, unsupported SVs often have unfavorable perceptions of their organizational culture.[12] When burdened with the emotional labor of a health care organization, the career trajectory as well as perceptions of the institution and its role can be altered.[18] Sexton and colleagues[5] reported those who lacked adequate institutional support had more negative impressions of the patient safety culture and well-being.

Although some organizations proclaim a no-blame and just culture, those involved in AE still express concerns about being blamed.[12] Managerial support is viewed as insincere and following procedures, expecting the HCWs to move forward from the event and deal with their emotions on their own.[12] Alternatively, those who turn to a peer have more positive impressions of the workplace culture than those who do not.[6]

RECOMMENDATIONS FOR SECOND-VICTIM SUPPORT

Following critical events what resources or support do SVs prefer? Some HCWs progress from the experience with adaptive skills[6,12] and favorable leadership support.[17,33] Alternatively, some HCWs view managerial support as lacking, insincere, unsupportive,[12,17] or failing to provide necessary guidance on investigative processes.[15] Chan and colleagues[15] reported that some HCWs chose personal self-determination, including religion to work through the experience; but some were hesitant to speak with unfamiliar individuals. Supporting SVs is the first line of preferred support (**Box 2**), and although this moral support can be offered by coworkers, managers, friends, or leaders,[17] a colleague is preferred·[16] and oftentimes utilized for support.[6] Studies reported that 69%[16] to 84%[8] desired a peer colleague.

In addition to the aforementioned preferred support of SVs, health care organizations have a pivotal role of placing high priority on safety culture, including an open and transparent environment, where high levels of shared beliefs by all on safety, values, and attitudes exist within the workplace.[1] In lieu of placing blame, the organization should maintain the privacy of all involved by upholding a nonpunitive environment and investigating systems failures that might have contributed to the AE.[17]

Following these processes, information can be shared among all HCWs in the hope of minimizing the risk of a similar event in the future. Information can flow via formal channels, including hospital websites, emails, meetings, group sessions, and notices about the AE, among others.[17] The limitations of sharing among such resources are assumptions the HCW is accessing these channels and reviewing.[17] Informal channels are often word of mouth among staff, which can advance rumors and criticism, or blame on the organization, negating a culture of safety.[17] Organizations should

---

Box 2
Desired support of second victims

Preferred Support

Peer support[6,8,16,33]

Time off[6–8,16]

Employee assistance programs[8,9,16,33]

Peaceful location to recover and recompose[8,16,33]

Conversations with manager/leader[6,8,16,17,33]

24-h access to talk with someone[8,16,33]

Time with counselor[8,16,33]

Openness and ability to talk about the event[10]

Moral and workload assistance from coworkers[17]

Empathy[9,17]

Leadership confidence in second victims[17]

Need for information[11]

Debrief[6]

---

communicate action plans and protocols following an AE to mitigate utilization of informal channels that often impede development of safety cultures.[17]

Finally, support program processes must be known to all[7]; an organization can have an abundance of resources to support SVs, but if there is a knowledge gap in accessing and utilizing these resources, efforts are futile. Draus[33] reported that 68.8% of SVs were unaware of any support resources. The Betsy Lehman report shares conflicting results between staff and leadership where almost 50% of staff and 67% of leaders were aware of the available support resources.[6] Sexton and colleagues[5] reported that 56.7% of management agreed that the SV receives institutional support, while only 31% of nurses and 24% of advanced practices providers agreed.

DISCUSSION

Since many HCWs electively choose health care professions due to compassion and desire to care for others, peer support programs are quite effective following exposures to AE.[6,8,16,33] Many HCWs who experience SVP turn to colleagues after an event (**Fig. 2**), but often, these encounters end before the SV has their emotional needs fully met.[2]

Prior to the organizational development of peer support teams to provide necessary and desired support, it is imperative the following actions first be implemented. When HCWs report inadequate institutional support, perceptions of safety culture are more negative.[5] A just culture for reporting AE and safe communication of lessons learned is a top priority, including confidentiality safeguards and protocols of peer and other emotional support interventions, as well as inclusivity of all involved in the event in debriefing, analysis, and sharing.[34]

Second, develop institution-wide campaigns to educate all on second-victim concepts and resources available;[2,33] otherwise, HCWs might be unaware of their existence.[33] Sharing clear instructions to all processes following AEs along with

OF STAFF WHO CONNECTED WITH SOMEONE, MOST
TALKED TO A PEER

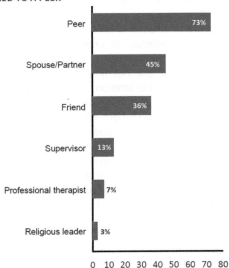

Fig. 2. Difficult events in patient care impact all staff, but support from peers can help, May 27, 2021. (*Reprinted with permission from* the Betsy Lehman Center for Patient Safety. Retrieved from https://betsylehmancenterma.gov/.)

expectations and responsibilities of the organization can possibly minimize confusion for SVs, with investigations and processes often foreign territory to many involved.[11,15]

Third, normalize second victimization and provide reassurance to the HCW that their emotions are normal responses.[9] Most SVs progress through similar stages of recovery, although the experiences of an SV can be unique to the individual. While an AE might be trivial to 1 HCW, a similar one may be devastating to another.[9] This can potentially mitigate stigma since some HCWs perceive reaching out will be viewed by others as a weakness and inability to perform their duties.[9] It must also be recognized some might not be impacted immediately following the event but later face the development of symptoms of SVP.[11]

Fourth, peer support programs should be voluntary; some might deem the event as not reaching a threshold to need support,[9] while others turn to external well-being habits.[6,9,12] Also, consideration for diversity among the peer support team, as second victimization does not discriminate based on gender,[2,8,10,13–16,21,33] age,[8,13,15,16,21,23,33] religion,[10,15] ethnicity,[10,16,23] education/professional status/job type,[2,5,6,8,10,13,14,21,23] or tenure.[2,5,8,11,13,15,16,23] Even those who are not directly involved in patient care are not immune.[5,6,8,23]

Finally, a follow-up from the peer supporter is desirable for continuity and to provide additional support if deemed appropriate by the SV.[9] In recognition of the limitations of a peer supporter's skills, knowledge of the availability of further resources must be inclusive of an organization's peer support program when an SV of distress warrants such support.[6,9,34]

SUMMARY

As health care providers, we strive for perfection; however, as humans, we do not exist in an infallible environment. It is a misfortune that AE and unexpected clinical events will plague those serving in organizations indefinitely, rendering one vulnerable to the SVP. Unfortunately, no HCW is immune and will likely experience this multiple times throughout a career.[6,8]

High-risk scenarios are multifactorial and include medical errors,[6,12] near misses,[8] pediatric patients,[24] patient deaths,[6] or any other challenging interaction or unexpected colleague event.[6]

Manifestations include (but are not limited to) physical, such as fatigue,[2,6,13] nausea,[16] insomnia,[2,6,12–16] muscle tension,[2,6] and hypertension.[2,13] Psychologically, SVs report depression,[2,10,13] scared,[14] lonely,[10,17] miserable,[16] relive the event,[2,6,10] and confusion and blame,[17] among others. Finally, professionally, there is worry about the future and being black-marked by peers,[15] decreased joy/meaning in work,[6,18] avoidance of patient care,[2] and social discrimination.[15] The recovery stages follow a predictable trajectory: chaos/event response, intrusive reflections, restoring personal integrity, enduring the inquisition, obtaining emotional first aid, and moving on.[2] Many report that following these occurrences, they became better providers[12,15,22] and eager to share their story to minimize the chance of a recurring event to their colleagues.[15]

Peer support and sharing the event with a colleague is one of many resources desired,[6,8,16,33] as well as time off,[6–8,16] speaking to a manager or leader,[6,8,16,17,33] and employee assistance programs.[8,9,16,33] It must be respected that peer support might not be desired by some[9] but, instead turn to adaptive coping mechanisms[6,12] or, perhaps their religious or spiritual beliefs.[15]

Health care organizations should advocate and implement a diverse array of resources to provide emotional support to SVs commencing with a just culture and transparency for reporting and learning from AEs.[34] Modeling this culture to all HCWs will promote changing the sense of loneliness[10] experienced by the SV to reassurance that the hospital will take care of them during stressful events.[7]

CLINICS CARE POINTS

- Second victimization occurs following AEs or wellness-related threats to all levels of HCWs.
- The physical, psychological, and professional or social manifestations can linger for extended periods of time.
- As one traverses through the recovery stages, adaptive and/or maladaptive coping mechanisms are utilized by HCWs.
- Health care organizations that implement and offer peer support programs to provide emotional support contribute to a culture of caring for SVs.

DISCLOSURE

The authors have no commercial associations that might pose a conflict of interest in connection with this work.

REFERENCES

1. Meyer WHOS. Patient Safety. Updated September 13, 2019 Available at: https://www.who.int/news-room/fact-sheets/detail/patient-safety. Accessed May 12, 2023.
2. Scott SD, Hirschinger LE, Cox KR, et al. The natural history of recovery for the healthcare provider "second victim" after adverse patient events. Qual Saf Health Care 2009;18(5):325–30.

3. Wu AW. Medical error: the second victim. The doctor who makes the mistake needs help too. Bmj 2000;320(7237):726–7.
4. Wu AW, Shapiro J, Harrison R, et al. The Impact of Adverse Events on Clinicians: What's in a Name? J Patient Saf 2020;16(1):65–72.
5. Sexton JB, Adair KC, Profit J, et al. Perceptions of Institutional Support for "Second Victims" Are Associated with Safety Culture and Workforce Well-Being. Jt Comm J Qual Patient Saf 2021;47(5):306–12.
6. Safety BLCfP. Difficult events in patient care impact all staff, but support from peers can help. Betsy Lehman Center for Patient Safety Available at: https://betsylehmancenterma.gov/news/difficult-events-in-patient-care-impact-all-staff-but-support-from-peers-can-help. Accessed May 27, 2023.
7. Cobos-Vargas A, Pérez-Pérez P, Núñez-Núñez M, et al. Second Victim Support at the Core of Severe Adverse Event Investigation. Int J Environ Res Publ Health 2022;(24):19.
8. Huang R, Sun H, Chen G, et al. Second-victim experience and support among nurses in mainland China. J Nurs Manag 2022;30(1):260–7.
9. Bakes-Denman L, Mansfield Y, Meehan T. Supporting mental health staff following exposure to occupational violence - staff perceptions of 'peer' support. Int J Ment Health Nurs 2021;30(1):158–66.
10. Amit Aharon A, Fariba M, Shoshana F, et al. Nurses as 'second victims' to their patients' suicidal attempts: A mixed-method study. J Clin Nurs 2021;30(21–22): 3290–300.
11. Kable A, Kelly B, Adams J. Effects of adverse events in health care on acute care nurses in an Australian context: A qualitative study. Nurs Health Sci 2018;20(2): 238–46.
12. Buhlmann M, Ewens B, Rashidi A. Moving on after critical incidents in health care: A qualitative study of the perspectives and experiences of second victims. J Adv Nurs 2022;78(9):2960–72.
13. Lang M, Jones L, Harvey C, et al. Workplace bullying, burnout and resilience amongst perioperative nurses in Australia: A descriptive correlational study. J Nurs Manag 2022;30(6):1502–13.
14. Sachdeva S, Jamshed N, Aggarwal P, et al. Perception of Workplace Violence in the Emergency Department. J Emerg Trauma Shock 2019;12(3):179–84.
15. Chan ST, Khong BPC, Pei Lin Tan L, et al. Experiences of Singapore nurses as second victims: A qualitative study. Nurs Health Sci 2018;20(2):165–72.
16. Mok WQ, Chin GF, Yap SF, et al. A cross-sectional survey on nurses' second victim experience and quality of support resources in Singapore. J Nurs Manag 2020;28(2):286–93.
17. Ferrús L, Silvestre C, Olivera G, et al. Qualitative Study About the Experiences of Colleagues of Health Professionals Involved in an Adverse Event. J Patient Saf 2021;17(1):36–43.
18. Rodriquez J, Scott SD. When clinicians drop out and start over after adverse events. Jt Comm J Qual Patient Saf 2018;44(3):137–45.
19. Occupational Safety and Health Administration. Workplace violence Available at: https://www.osha.gov/workplace-violence. Accessed September 9, 2023.
20. Al-Qadi MM. Workplace violence in nursing: A concept analysis. J Occup Health 2021;63(1):e12226.
21. Xu H, Cao X, Jin QX, et al. Distress, support and psychological resilience of psychiatric nurses as second victims after violence: A cross-sectional study. J Nurs Manag 2022;30(6):1777–87.

22. Foli KJ, Forster A, Cheng C, et al. Voices from the COVID-19 frontline: Nurses' trauma and coping. J Adv Nurs 2021;77(9):3853–66.
23. Mental Health America. The mental health of healthcare workers. A survey of concerns and needs of frontline workers as the pandemic enters its third year Available at: https://mhanational.org/research-reports/healthcare-workers. Accessed September 9, 2023.
24. Agency for Healthcare Research and Quality. The Second Victim Phenomenon: A Harsh Reality of Health Care Professions. May 1, 2011 Available at: https://psnet.ahrq.gov/perspective/second-victim-phenomenon-harsh-reality-health-care-professions. Accessed June 25, 2023.
25. National Library for Medicine. Depression: What is burnout?. June 18, 2020 Available at: https://www.ncbi.nlm.nih.gov/books/NBK279286/. Accessed July 2, 2023.
26. World Health Organization. Burn-out an "occupational phenomenon": International classifications of diseases Available at: https://www.who.int/news/item/28-05-2019-burn-out-an-occupational-phenomenon-international-classification-of-diseases. Accessed September 9, 2023.
27. Tawfik DS, Profit J, Morgenthaler TI, et al. Physician Burnout, Well-being, and Work Unit Safety Grades in Relationship to Reported Medical Errors. Mayo Clin Proc 2018;93(11):1571–80.
28. Nursing shortage fact sheet. American Association of Colleges of Nursing. October 2022 Available at: https://www.aacnnursing.org/news-data/fact-sheets/nursing-shortage. Accessed September 9, 2023.
29. Nurse.com. Nurse salary research report 2022 Available at: https://www.nurse.com/nursing-salary-research-report. Accessed September 9, 2023.
30. Burlison JD, Quillivan RR, Scott SD, et al. The Effects of the Second Victim Phenomenon on Work-Related Outcomes: Connecting Self-Reported Caregiver Distress to Turnover Intentions and Absenteeism. J Patient Saf 2021;17(3):195–9.
31. Institute for Healthcare Improvement. The IHI triple aim Available at: https://www.ihi.org/Engage/Initiatives/TripleAim/Pages/default.aspx#:~:text=Improving%20the%20patient%20experience%20of,capita%20cost%20of%20health%20care. Accessed September 9, 2023.
32. Sikka R, Morath JM, Leape L. The Quadruple Aim: care, health, cost and meaning in work. BMJ Qual Saf 2015;24:608–10.
33. Draus C, Mianecki TB, Musgrove H, et al. Perceptions of Nurses Who Are Second Victims in a Hospital Setting. J Nurs Care Qual 2022;37(2):110–6.
34. The Joint Commission. Supporting second victims Available at: https://www.jointcommission.org/resources/news-and-multimedia/newsletters/newsletters/quick-safety/quick-safety-issue-39-supporting-second-victims/. Accessed July 20, 2023.

9780443130076